P9-CSC-127

Shameless

Shameless

How I ditched the diet, got naked, found true pleasure . . . and somehow got home in time to cook dinner

Pamela Madsen

with

Anne Adams

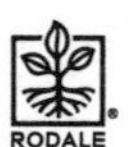

Rodale books may be purchased for business or promotional use or for special sales. For information, please write to: Special Markets Department, Rodale Inc., 733 Third Avenue, New York, NY 10017.

Printed in the United States of America

Rodale Inc. makes every effort to use acid-free ♾, recycled paper ♻.

Book design by Sara Stemen

Library of Congress Cataloging-in-Publication Data

Madsen, Pamela.
Shameless : how I ditched the diet, got naked, found true pleasure . . . and somehow got home in time to cook dinner / Pamela Madsen.
p. cm.
ISBN 978-1-60529-175-8 hardcover
1. Madsen, Pamela. 2. Sex therapy. 3. Women—Sexual behavior. I. Title.
RC557.M33 2011
616.85'8306092—dc22 2010047723

Distributed to the trade by Macmillan

2 4 6 8 10 9 7 5 3 1 hardcover

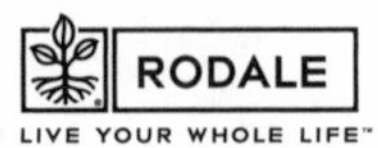

www.rodalebooks.com

Early in my odyssey to Shameless, *I realized my path was made easier by the standing, often-battered army of sexual theorists, practitioners, explorers, and teachers who openly and brazenly worked to demystify sexuality. Without their determination to integrate this most fundamental of human needs into daily life, I'd never have had the courage or a place to start, let alone succeed. Thank you all.*

You know who you are.

And the day came when the risk to remain tight in a bud was more painful than the risk it took to blossom.

—Anaïs Nin

Contents

Chapter 1: A Seismic Shift 1

Chapter 2: She's Not Who She Seems 15

Chapter 3: A Massage By Any Other Name 21

Chapter 4: Outside My Box 25

Chapter 5: Move Over, Pussy Galore 31

Chapter 6: Birth of an Everyday Supergoddess, or, First You Ask Your Son 41

Chapter 7: If I Was a Gay Man, Ya Ha Deedle Deedle, Bubba Bubba Deedle Deedle Dum 49

Chapter 8: Queens and Tigers and Pam, Oh My 57

Chapter 9: The Year of the Tiger 65

Chapter 10: Home Again 73

Chapter 11: An Unexpected Geisha 77

Chapter 12: She Wore a Raspberry Beret 83

Chapter 13: Homework 87

Chapter 14: Rockin' It at Babeland 93

Chapter 15: Crazy Fruit Salad 103

Chapter 16: Between Rock and My G-Spot 109

Chapter 17: Here's to You, Mrs. Robinson 115

Chapter 18: A Ripe Piece of Melon 119

CONTENTS

Chapter 19: Fantasies Unveiled ... 123

Chapter 20: Okay! I Admit It! I Shop at Chico's ... 131

Chapter 21: The Red Shoe Diaries ... 137

Chapter 22: When Worlds Collide ... 149

Chapter 23: Fearing the Scarlet Letter ... 155

Chapter 24: Goddess in Green Cellophane ... 159

Chapter 25: Women Loving Women ... 165

Chapter 26: A New Hankering ... 173

Chapter 27: Celebrating the Body Erotic ... 179

Chapter 28: My Big Fat Lesbian Experience ... 189

Chapter 29: One Last Bridge ... 193

Chapter 30: Purple Passion ... 203

Chapter 31: Letting Gavin See ... 213

Chapter 32: Motherload ... 221

Chapter 33: The Kinky Daughter and the Jewish Mother ... 227

Chapter 34: And Now for Something Completely Different ... 233

Chapter 35: Power, Surrender, and Intimacy: The Dark Knight ... 241

Chapter 36: Mistress Beth ... 251

Chapter 37: Long Live Love in Leather ... 257

Chapter 38: Goddess Lost ... 263

Chapter 39: Who Makes the Rules, Anyway? ... 269

Epilogue ... 273

Acknowledgments ... 277

Chapter One

A Seismic Shift

Funny how things that change overnight often are years in the making. Earthquakes, for instance. Plates deep beneath the surface move, shift, bump, and grind for eons. All that subterranean action sends up warning tremors, little rumbles that are often too small to notice. Until the big one hits, the one that shatters windows, brings down buildings, and snaps bridges in two.

I am an earthquake.

The first obvious tremblers hit when I corralled my Martini Gang—my sister, my cousin on my mother's side, and my two best girlfriends—into an "authentic" Korean spa for a day of tubs, scrubs, and hot-crystal meditation rooms. I'd read about it in the *New York Times* months before. It sounded fabulous. Wrangling all of us into the same place at the same time, however, was not so fabulous. It required weeks of intense negotiations. I got less agitated bringing a nonprofit staff and a board of directors into agreement on a radical new fertility policy than I got pulling five of us together. Even for a self-made, headstrong executive director like me, nothing's harder than coordinating type-A women who are overextended with work, children, and some version of a marriage. Especially when it involves them abandoning their homesteads early on a summer Sunday for exotic indulgences beyond the Manhattan city limits in Fort Lee, New Jersey.

Beth was the special challenge. Her life had more moving parts than a pinball machine. I knew she had to wrestle with her volatile brood of four adolescent girls, the dog, the garden, the twenty-year marriage, and, of course, the boyfriend. She ran a small, well-curated art gallery and indiscriminately served on do-gooder committees. The two E's were her constants: Erratic schedules and Emergencies.

I maneuvered into a parking space next to Beth's eco-friendly hybrid. She had arrived seconds before me and was leaning against her car, long black hair blowing in the Sahara-like wind, deep in an animated phone conversation. Two minutes later, Vicki—my big sister—pulled in behind me. She had Cousin Sophia, my own personal Italian-Jewish Auntie Mame, in tow. Vicki locked up and they walked over, Sophia carrying off the billowy chiffon top that hid her lovely roundness and made her seem much younger than her sixty-plus years.

"Husband or Kevin?" Vicki asked, raising an artfully shaped eyebrow.

Beth snapped the cell phone shut. Her flushed cheeks were a dead giveaway. I knew that look. I knew everything about her since we were five years old and our mothers made us hold hands the first time we went ice-skating. We haven't let go since. Beth put on oversized shades to hide her obviously teary brown eyes. Loverland isn't always easy.

"Kevin," Vicki and I chorused softly.

"Did you tell Mom what we were doing today?" I asked Vicki while we waited for Beth to compose herself.

"Absolutely not!" Vicki was vehement.

"So neither one of us checked in. . . . That's going to go over really well."

"I coulda been lyin' dead on the floor for all anyone would know. What would it take? One phone call?" Vicki's Mom schtick was dead-on. She was a carbon copy of our mother, right down to the curve of her long, shapely legs.

We burst out laughing.

"Just the idea of your tennis-playing, step-dancing, aquasizing eighty-year-old mother helpless anywhere is just too funny. Aunt Roz would love to be here, a day with the girls," Sophia said.

"Ooh, that would have been perfect. Why didn't I think of that?" I said, my conscience kicking in. "Damn it. I'll call her on the way home and take the hit."

Beth waved her hand to get our attention, as if we weren't standing an unobstructed five feet away. She craned her neck, scouring the crowd. "Let me guess, Olivia's not here yet."

We loitered in the sticky tar parking lot, pale Amazons in a sea of tiny Korean women all headed for the King Spa. Olivia was always punctually ten minutes late. Her computer went down. Her genius twin boys were one chemical compound away from a patentable cure for carbohydrate cravings. Her petulance-prone lover threatened suicide if she did not leave her husband. Dire or magnificent, the issue always took Olivia an unscheduled ten minutes to resolve. It made her even more exotic than her half-Chinese and half–European Jewish one-of-a-kind beauty. She loved signing her e-mails "*xoxo your Chinkajew.*"

At precisely 10:10, she arrived. She waved a languid hello, parked, and joined us on our pilgrimage past the roasting cars to the bland seventies industrial warehouse. We squeezed in a huddle around the shoulder-high reception desk, firing way too many questions.

What exactly is a face-whitening facial? Could we get five salt scrubs at the same time? And the foot reflexology, too? What do you mean these wristbands track what we spend?

"For chrissakes, just pay and go in," snapped the woman behind us. I wheeled around with a ready retort, but then I saw the pileup behind us. The crowd was turning ugly.

"Sorry, sorry. Really sorry," the five of us called to the surging throng, throwing credit cards at the cashier.

In return we were handed the most god-awful gym outfits ever. We went to Dressing Room 1, where we ditched our street clothes and slipped into the mandatory uni-"sexless" Pepto-pink spa wear required for the coed areas. The color didn't work for me, but I was thrilled to feel diminutive in the "one size fits pretty much everyone on earth" getup. The best part—there were no pockets. No pockets meant no cell phones. Nobody—not work, the kids, my husband, or even my mother—could reach me for hours.

A thick glass wall separated the changing area from the bathhouse, a space so beautiful and strange, it stopped us dead in our tracks. It wasn't the immaculate elegance of the glass-and-stone-tile spa that got us. It wasn't the gargantuan hot, cold, and warm tubs; frigid open showers; or the sauna and steam rooms that knocked us out. It was the vision of dozens of naked women squatting at handheld shower stations scrubbing their most intimate anatomy with abandon, washing each other's backs, butts, breasts, and whatnots.

"Whoa! Now, that's different," Beth muttered in my ear. "Did the *Times* article say anything about that?"

"Looks great!" Vicki said. My brave sister was always up for anything. "Who wants to wash my pits?"

We stripped down to nothing in the locker room. Vicki strutted by with her new, postcancer rebuilt breasts. There was no way I could avoid them or the mortality that hovered over my once-invincible sister. These breasts were huge, two Pamela Anderson–sized mountains with riverbed scars running along their sides and bottoms.

"You could clean up on the strip circuit with those," I said, batting away the powerful combination of awe and upset with a one-liner. It was shocking to see that her breasts dwarfed mine when I had always been at least one cup size bigger, the one thing I inherited from my mother that she didn't.

"Yeah, it's bizarre. Men trip over themselves looking at these babies." Her wan smile turned into an angry pout. "I told that doctor to keep them the way they were. What is it with men? They want every woman to have gigantic hooters; therefore we must want them, too? I hate the surgeon. I told him to keep them small. But no-o-o. Now I'm stuck with these."

"Well, honey, they're magnificent," I soothed her.

"You really think so?" Vicki was still insecure after a double mastectomy, reconstructive surgery, and a couple of life-threatening infections over the past year. It was a miracle that we were standing here together.

We followed Beth, Sophia, and Olivia through the door to the spa. I lagged behind my sisterhood of four, watching their curvaceous bodies and round asses sway, hands fluttering as they brought each other up to date. I waded slowly into the hottest of the tubs, a large, shallow, blue-tiled pool ringed with at least a dozen women and girls, not one larger than my thigh. I settled near a jet and cooked. One by one, Vicki, Beth, Sophia, and Olivia joined me with the requisite "Argh! It's ho-o-ot. Oh, man! Ahhh, that's good!"

We found five spots together, and chatted about everyday work/kid stuff. This was always the prelude to the heavier subjects.

"You be quiet here. This peaceful place." A deep voice made us leap like startled fish. A burly bathhouse attendant loomed over us, her eyes stern with authority. "And you! You put up your hair!" She thrust rubber bands at Olivia, Beth, and me. Resentfully, Olivia piled her chestnut hair into a messy bun on top of her head; Beth and I followed her lead. Hair up, voices down. That lasted for about thirty seconds.

"Ya think we stand out enough?" Vicki said in her best Bronx honk. What didn't she inherit from our mother?

"Nah, we blend right in," I countered, glancing down at my ample C-cup breasts bobbing, cocking my head at the training bra–sized boobs of the dozen other boiling women and their offspring.

"One wrong move and my butt could cause some serious injury. I never saw so many small-boned people," Beth whispered.

"Maybe we should find a quieter corner," Olivia suggested. She looked me over as I stood up. "We sure have come a long way since I first interviewed you all those years ago. I'm so relieved I'm off the fertility beat. It broke my heart every time I produced one of those segments."

"At least you got me out of it," I answered. "Didn't that make working in daytime TV worthwhile?"

"So totally," she giggled, splashing water at me.

We trooped over to the uninhabited tepid tub, plunging back into the conversation the second we settled.

For me, it was an extension of the daily check-ins I had with Vicki and Olivia. Sophia called once every week or two. Beth was a different story altogether. We talked somewhere between two and fifty times a day, as we had for decades. It was like my ear had sprouted a blinking Bluetooth. I talked while doing the laundry, getting fresh produce, or trekking from fertility centers to pharmaceutical companies, making the fertility patient advocacy pitch. We craved the connection that some scientists say is a uniquely feminine thing. I think it's just human.

I was ready with my "back on Atkins—I have to lose sixty pounds—women are so screwed" rap when Beth usurped my place.

"I got the most amazing head last week," she burst out, totally smug.

Oh no she didn't! She'd switched up the order of our traditional agenda: weight and body image first, then sex. I looked to Sophia to put a stop to this. She was, after all, the grande dame of the group, our resident moderator. She rolled her eyes but didn't rescue me.

"Let me guess. It was Kevin. I'll bet my last paycheck it wasn't Larry," I snapped, my guts in a sudden uproar. This was a sex-talk ambush. I had to warm up before I could listen to her gush about the unbridled pleasure of her lover working away between her legs. I needed conversational foreplay. Beth met Kevin over free-range eggs at a food co-op a couple of years ago. Who knew organic groceries were an aphrodisiac? I'd been listening to her talk about him every day since. I saw him once getting out of a car, and that was close enough for me. None of us wanted to socialize with anybody's lover. It was enough to talk about them in excruciating detail.

Besides, it wasn't about a particular lover. It was about my friends dealing with the various stages of disgust, heartbreak, and *finito* with their marriages. Husbands who couldn't or wouldn't meet them where they were, as they were, now. Two of them found refuge in extramarital affairs. Vicki was seriously flirting with the idea, her discontent heightened by her brush with death.

Sophia, on the other hand, never stayed in a marriage long enough to have an affair. So she said.

Beth was unstoppable. "Well, Kev is fantastic. He loves women's bodies. He spends hours romancing the vulva."

Blech. I slid down and let the embryonic water cover my ears. I could still hear every word. They were sending out sex vibes that the water amplified until they were like shock waves. I felt them trigger an internal seismic upheaval I didn't understand. Usually our girl-time was a no-holds-barred free-for-all that I treasured. Why the talk today was provoking an anxiety attack was beyond me. But it was.

"I'm hungry," I announced, standing up fast enough to send waves crashing over the sides. "The *Times* said the food upstairs is delish—lots of protein and cabbage. Perfect for Atkins, which I'm back on, in case anybody is interested."

But before I could even step out of the tub, Vicki chimed in.

"I can remember what that felt like. I still get that shiver when I run into some guy and the electricity starts running like crazy. I just don't have the patience to do anything about it. Yet." Vicki completely ignored my plea for kimchi. Olivia nodded in recognition. Her husband was brilliant, but a social nerd. Her boyfriend wasn't quite as smart, but he crackled with a crazy sexual energy and street smarts that turned her on. And that turned the always private, prim Olivia into a wild woman. She didn't talk about it much, but when she did, I could see her on the back of Colin's Harley, her thighs gripping his from behind. I didn't wait around for her to paint the image. I heaved myself out of the tub, almost falling down on the slippery tile. "I'm going upstairs to get a table," I said. I wrapped myself in the complimentary micro-mini-towel and stormed back to the dressing room.

I had been feeling uneasy since the night before. My youngest son, Ben, had found my dust-covered wedding album on the top shelf of our living room entertainment center. He pulled it down and started leafing through it, asking for the names of all the dead relatives. I sat on the couch next to him and annotated my ancient wedding party. He and I looked at the pictures of the slender, twenty-year-old bride and her fresh-faced groom. "Mom, you look like you were Andrew's age when you got married." He was stunned that I was ever that young.

"Well, I was only a couple of years older than Andrew, but I was even younger than he is now when I met Daddy. I was a mere seventeen on the cusp of eighteen."

I told Ben the familiar story of "how Daddy and I met" during my senior year at the Village School in Great Neck. I was a reporter on the school paper doing my version of an investigative piece on the Merchant Marine Academy at Kings Point, a mysterious military college full of "older" men in uniform. It was a place where good girls didn't venture.

"Really, it was my chance to go meet 'An Officer and a Gentleman'—you remember the Richard Gere movie. It was a big hit right around then and I must have seen it three times. And look what happened. Two years later we got married under a cross of swords. Hollywood had nothing on us."

"You were twenty? That's only five years older than me!" He paused. "Did you ever have any other serious boyfriends?"

My voiced cracked. "Nope, Ben, he was and is my one and only."

"Aw," Ben said, punching my shoulder affectionately. "That's so sweet. None of my friend's parents have been together that long."

Sweet. That's what everyone said. High school sweethearts, how unusual. And under the cooing was always a little bit of surprise and the unspoken question: How is it possible to be faithful to one person for that long?

Lately, I couldn't help wondering: Did it make me some sort of freak? Is that why I was feeling so set apart from my friends? They all had rich lover histories. Now, with their extramarital activities, it was like they were stoned on something that I never got a chance to smoke. Even Vicki, still (reluctantly) faithful to her husband, seemed alive with sex. Marrying the person you lost your virginity to, as I had, seemed almost antiquated, a story from the nineteenth century.

Thumbing through my wedding album with Ben, I felt newly self-conscious about my life, unexpectedly restless, and that pissed me off. I was successful by any measure. I was a prominent patient advocate, damn it, regularly interviewed by the national media. I cooked and shopped, and I mothered two clever, sturdy boys. Maybe now that I had done it all, built the family and the organization, I finally had enough time to stop running and just feel. Sure, there had always been the vaguest hint of envy when the girls ran on about their escapades, but I hadn't had a second to give it any thought.

Besides, I loved my husband. My beautiful husband. We were true life partners. I opened new worlds to him—fatherhood, friends, and travel. He was my ground control, the perfect helpmate for a woman with a full-time, slightly off-the-charts life. He generously pitched in without ever complaining. I thought he was handsome. He thought I was gorgeous, even if I didn't. We were a well-oiled marriage machine. I thought we had it all. So why was I suddenly shaking with discontent? What the hell was missing?

I was marooned in the spa's giant dining hall, stranded in an ocean of wholesome families dressed in the same hide-your-gender outfits, when it hit me. Sex. Steamy and luscious sex. Sex like I hadn't had in I don't know how long. I couldn't even remember the last time I truly wanted hot, steamy sex.

Even when I was a head-turner back in the day, I'd never experienced raw sexuality and freedom. I never dared express the torrid passions that drove my friends into their lovers' beds, my sister to distraction in her flatlining marriage, and that made my cousin shy of long-term monogamy. The hot tub melted the remnants of the everyday busyness and success I used as my shield against self-knowledge. I'd invested a lot in the fairy tale of my life and here it was, dripping off me like the sweat running down my face.

Beth, Vicki, Sophia, and Olivia radiated sensual heat, while I radiated competence. If I was going to be truthful with myself, I had to admit that lately their sex rants sparked a deep-down ache that forced me to acknowledge my own discontent. Until now I'd done a masterful job of squashing the urge for anything other than what Gavin and I had when we rubbed up against each other. But an unnamed desire was there—rumbling, insistent, impolite, and, scariest of all, bubbling toward the surface.

"You ordah?" The genial guy behind the counter looked at me expectantly. "You ordah?" he asked again, waiting for me to pick from the incomprehensible menu hanging above his head.

"I want the bibimbap," Vicki brayed. I jumped out of my skin. The girls had snuck up behind me on little spa feet.

"I'll have the chicken soup with the chestnut thing. I always need hot soup," Olivia said, delicate yet decisive. The way Olivia always picked at her food to maintain her birdlike frame bugged the shit out of me. Two bites were a meal.

"I want that too. And whatever that fruit thing is," added Beth, impolitely pointing to an elaborate dish weighing down a nearby table. What was even more annoying than watching Olivia starve herself was that Beth could eat me under the table, complain about her weight, and still attain a yoga-hard body, even if there was more heft than when she was eighteen and a size 4. I hated them.

"That's mostly water," I piped up. "That'll go through us in an hour. We need protein." Always a proponent of overordering, I reeled off the meatiest-sounding dishes.

"Too much! Too much!" The guy behind the counter cut me off just as I hit my stride.

"Too much for whom? Five New York women on diets? You gotta be kidding," I mumbled, taking the number he shoved at me to identify the table of the bottomless pits.

A few minutes later, a petite waitress dragged over another table to hold the countless steaming plates. We dug in with gusto. Before I could swallow the first mouthful, they picked up the conversation right where I bailed. I almost choked.

"Sometimes I think Colin has actually changed my chemistry." With her blood sugar now stabilized, Olivia was perking up. "I can't ever remember feeling this good in my body. I mean, he knows exactly what to do and how to keep it going. He's . . ." With characteristic witchery, Olivia trained her gray, almond-shaped eyes on me. "Pammy, what's the matter? Are you okay?" I was a second away from a cloudburst, face bright red and neck swollen with frustration. I dissolved over the spicy tofu stew.

"I don't know," I croaked. It was so humiliating, but if I couldn't tell them, whom could I tell?

"I feel trapped in my own life. I listen to you guys, all 'Woohoo. Look at me. I'm a sex goddess.' Well, I'm not. I'm a bundle of missed opportunities."

Sophia put a steadying hand on my arm to keep me from flying apart. "Pammy, honey. What're you talking about?"

"You guys have been playing the field since you were, what, twelve? I've been with Gavin since before I was legal. I saved myself for him, as if saving myself for marriage earned me some kind of merit badge. Well, it's been a fucking quarter of a fucking century and the badge is rusty. You know? There's so much I never felt. So much I'm never gonna know."

Vicki wrapped a big-sister arm around my shoulder. "C'mon, Pammy. What you and Gavin have is so sweet. Like, how many people do we know who have been that loyal to each other?"

"My freakish monogamy again? Don't give me 'sweet.' How many times have you all asked me how I stand it? Well, to tell you the truth, I'm tired of pretending that it's enough. And that makes me feel rotten. I don't want to have an affair. It won't work for me. None of you was a virgin when you got married. You have no idea how loaded that is for Gavin and me. It's a point of pride, a sacred covenant. It's not something I would breach. But I feel jealous of you. I want something else."

I turned to Beth. "You talk about Kevin and it takes you somewhere I've never been. I want to go there, too, but the thought of it scares the crap out of me. . . . I just don't want to die without feeling another man's hands on my body."

I slurped another giant spoonful of tofu stew. Emotion tended to accelerate my rate of consumption.

This was the first time I had ever copped to feeling the same yearning they did, and they looked at me with surprise, concern, and sympathy. I'd always been such a Freudian caricature, rebelling against my oh-so-liberated family. Vicki and our much older brother had pot and sex parties every time our parents went on a business trip, and they called it babysitting. My parents weren't any better. They'd come back from Europe or Latin America ripe with tales of lusty nights. To this day, Mom keeps the silver-framed picture of my father prancing around in her green and white striped panties one crazy night in Rio. What a renegade I was—making a stand as Great Neck, Long Island's, only Jewish vestal virgin.

Olivia opened her huge eyes wider and threw down a dare. "So, Pam, you want another man's hands? Go find 'em."

"And then what?"

My mind was racing, my stomach let loose a bowel-deep yelp for help. We sat paralyzed until I unleashed an incongruously little earthquake of a belch. When those tectonic plates move, you can't fight 'em.

"Too much kimchi," Vicki offered.

Nope, it was a sign. Something had shifted. I just wasn't sure what. In the meantime, there was always food. "Beth, you gonna eat that rice?" I asked. They all shoved their plates in my direction.

Chapter Two

She's Not Who She Seems

My confession left me raw. I had said it out loud. I brought a dark secret out into the light and I wasn't dead. Nothing perceptibly changed, except the next few days my cranky quotient was way up. Yeah, yeah, I loved Gavin. But I was picking on him the way you pick lice out of your kid's hair.

"What's so hard about trimming your nails?" Who was that bitch? Me? "Your feet look like they belong to a troll." I cast a withering glance at the curling talons.

"Well, I can't find the clippers. Somebody's always moving them."

I stomped over to the dresser drawer that had held the famous disappearing clippers for the last fifteen years, pulled out two pairs, and hurled them across the room.

Despite the clinging funk, we managed our usual "Swanson TV Dinner" sex that night. We waited until Ben and Andrew retreated to their room, the only real bedroom in our apartment, so that Gavin and I could go at it with muted pleasure in the dining alcove that we had converted into our sleeping capsule. It was a predictable, enjoyable release. We slept entwined.

The next morning the aftershocks of the spa disclosure were coming fast and furious. It was hard to concentrate on work. My organization's health fair at the Grand Hyatt was only six months away and I still hadn't locked down the details. Some executive director I was. I called the hotel's catering manager and left a message telling her I'd be by later that day. I needed to focus.

Bitsy, a longtime volunteer at the organization and a close friend, agreed to come along. I was pacing outside waiting for her when her Mercedes silently rolled up on the pavement, missing my foot by a couple of inches.

"Wanna drive?" she asked, the window still mostly closed. As usual, she wore her long, unruly red hair in a tight bun at the nape of her neck; it looked especially bright against the dark leather interior of the car. She offered because I'd told her how much I loved getting behind the wheel of her gazillion-dollar baby, which was partly true. The other ninety percent of the reason was her driving. It was awful, hair-raising, death defying. I'd promised Gavin I'd never let her chauffeur me anywhere, especially after the DMV revoked her E-Z Pass for speeding through the tolls. Looking at Bitsy, in her overpriced gray cashmere knits, you'd never know she had a reckless streak.

"Yeah," I answered, the lack of enthusiasm obvious. I took over like I was doing her a big favor.

"Pamela. Yoo-hoo. You there?"

"Just tired." She could tell that I was withholding something. I wasn't up for the big reveal. She didn't press. When I first met her at a women's fertility support group, I never could have imagined how deep our friendship would grow. It seemed like Bitsy, partial to demure pearls, sensible heels, and meticulous manners, wouldn't have much in common with a devotee of chunky turquoise pieces, cowboy boots, and boisterous good times. Yet it was me she trusted with coordinating the burial of her influential husband, Howard, five years ago. I had held her literally and figuratively for months, at my house or hers, while she nearly drowned in the perfect storm of grief and anger that comes with an unexpected death.

I had never liked Howard. He treated Bitsy, and everyone around her, like shit. Howard even had the balls to blame her for their infertility when nobody could figure out what the problem was. After years of grueling treatment, she had finally delivered a daughter, Karina, and he bitched that she wasn't a boy. Still, Bitsy took her identity from being the wife of a powerbroker and she lost all her bearings when he died. Since Howard's (some would say) untimely death, Bitsy had become part of my family.

I got us to the Grand Hyatt in record time through the congested midtown Manhattan traffic, with Bitsy speed-talking the way she did when she was pent up.

"So I'm going to try eHarmony. I've been thinking about it and you're right. I need to go out, see what other men are like."

"This is good, Bits," I said. "I'm proud of you."

I drove right up to a rare metered space a couple of blocks from the hotel. I was backing into it when a Lexus full of suburban ladies out for the day pulled nose-first into our spot. Before I could stop her, Bitsy was out of the car, menacing them with a diamond-studded fist.

"You fucking better be careful," Bitsy screamed. "You don't know who my husband is. You're walking into a world of hurt."

Bitsy Soprano! She scared even me—and I knew her husband was dead. Beneath the silk, Bits had some of the sharpest edges I'd ever come up against. The Lexus skidded away.

Inside the frigid hotel lobby, however, Bitsy became all business. "Pamela Madsen and Bitsy Sullivan. We're here for a meeting with Bonnie White, the event manager," she informed the concierge.

"She's waiting for you in the Blue Room."

I turned and whispered, "Good thing you didn't have to kill those women, Bits. The whole jail thing would have made us so tardy."

"I know." Bitsy's hangdog look was kind of adorable, her blush rising to her hairline. "I do have to watch that temper of mine."

Ms. White took us through the tasting ritual, assuring us our health fair would be "truly fantastic," then sat us down in a corner of the lobby to review the contracts.

It was impossible to concentrate. I was becoming sex obsessed. My brain was turning into a bodice-ripper on steroids. Every passing man was a romance novel waiting to happen. Gorgeous, buff guys in $2,000 suits and with $200 haircuts who could easily seduce—dancing at the Rainbow Room, gift boxes filled with handmade lace teddies that they'd want me to wear just for them. There was this one "aw shucks" cowboy with worn jeans and a tight butt. I could feel his arms sweep me up onto the back of his wild mustang. Could they smell my pheromones? I never let my mind wander these fields, but I couldn't stop it. I hadn't experienced anything like this in more than twenty-five years, not since the first of my two pre-Gavin "boyfriends." I remembered having an unchained libido. I made out; I went to second base in the woods, in the living room, behind the high school, in the back of the bus on the class trip. By the time I met Gavin, I could hardly wait to go all the way. We couldn't hold out until the wedding, but we managed until my eighteenth birthday. Ever since then, we've had good sex (not that I would know any different). I've had sex on my side, on my knees, from the front, and from behind. He was never shy about putting his mouth anywhere. What else was there?

That's the question that had me squeezing my legs together in the lobby, window-shopping. I was off my rocker. My frisky inner fifteen-year-old was banging on the bars and howling.

"Pam!" Bitsy was brusque. "The contract looks fine. Let's just sign. I'm late for a meeting with Karina's therapist. What is up with you today?"

"Okay, okay. I'm scheduled for a massage anyway. I'll sign, you can go. Really, I'll take care of the rest."

She sailed off in a cloud of Patou's Joy. I waded through the sea of testosterone to the exit. Every time I made eye contact, I was certain each guy knew exactly what I was thinking. I was positive that guy in handmade cowboy boots had just winked.

Chapter Three

A Massage By Any Other Name

Damp with sinful imaginings and Big Apple humidity, I couldn't wait to get out of the lobby and into a cab. Mercifully, the low lights, scented candles, and plinking lute music of the Zen room in a posh East Side hotel spa triggered a Pavlovian reaction. I went on autopilot, stripping and clambering up on the cool sheets of the massage table. I'd been doing this for four years with Ricky. Our routine—the waiting hot spiced tea, cold cucumber water, and plush terry-cloth robe—was the only full stop in my go-go life.

Ricky burst in. He was wired. That was part of the routine, too. We were way past the "Good afternoon, Mrs. Madsen. How are we today?" phase.

He started right in with his usual dish about sexcapades in the gay world. Mostly, Ricky's ramblings were amusing white noise. Once in a while, I egged him on between breaths. Usually, they were all fantasies anyway. Today I just wasn't in the mood. Oblivious to my indifference, he let it rip.

"Pammy, I swear, it was just what I needed to take the edge off. It was the best massage, a nice little erotic recharge. You know, I do love my hubby, but sometimes our sex feels so . . . " Ricky's professional whisper trailed off into loaded silence. He recovered quickly. "I mean, it's been seven years. My massage therapist was adorable and I got up off the table feeling so much better. I actually couldn't wait to get home to see my honey."

His words yanked me back from the depths of semiconsciousness so fast I almost got the bends. Did he say "erotic" and "massage" in the same sentence? Excuse me? In my next life I'm so coming back as a gay man.

I sat bolt upright, clocking Ricky in the jaw with an audible crack. "Omigod, Ricky. Are you okay?"

I looked for signs of concussion. Both pupils seemed roughly the same. "You're fine. Now, what was that about your massage and your hubby? Does he know? Does he do this? How come you never told me about this before, you dirty holdout. What, I'm chopped liver?"

"No, he doesn't know. And if you meet him, don't you dare say a word. And no, I don't think he uses these services. He better not! But sometimes I feel trapped by my marriage, Pammy, and I have to do something. I don't want to cheat on him. I certainly don't want to fall in love with someone else. So I make an appointment with a cute guy who's a pro at erotic massage. An hour and a half later, I'm good to go. It's simple, safe, and uncomplicated."

"I don't get it. How is this not cheating? If it's really not, why haven't you told your honey?"

Ricky grew thoughtful. "I don't want Mitch to think that he doesn't make me happy. He does. It's not that. It's about me, my needs, my desires, my body. With my pro, I don't have to worry about satisfying him. I just get touched, like you are now. You don't worry about my feelings, you simply pay me. It's exactly like that."

I chewed on this. Ricky had hit upon the perfect solution. Fee-for-service and one-way touch kept his boundaries intact.

Maybe it was my perfect solution, too. It sounded so logical, so delicious. My flesh quivered with possibility. I'd heard about "happy ending" massages. Who hadn't? But until Ricky, I'd thought it was an urban legend. I didn't know anyone who'd actually had one. Were there such things for women? The idea was intoxicating: ninety sensually charged minutes with no emotional complications and my virtue unscathed.

I stumbled out of Ricky's Zen room into another taxi for the ride home. My phone twittered with Gavin's special ring.

"How's my girl?" he chirped into my ear. "Do we need anything?"

It was as regular as the sun setting. He made that call every day before heading home from the office. He'd pick up milk, eggs, cheese, or bread. It didn't matter how tired he was or what kind of day he'd had. For my part, I made sure there would be something tasty bubbling on the stove, a stocked refrigerator, and clean laundry waiting for him. We had our undeclared, cherished rituals.

"We have everything that we need, honey. Just come home."

"Okeydoke. . . ."

It was such a simple thing, such a display of love. I adored my Gavin, and I felt devoted to my devoted husband. But that was my marriage. I wanted sensual massage. Two completely different animals. The more I thought about it, the more doable it seemed. The very notion of a contained erotic escape flickered like a bright light in the dark. There was a way to get man hands, after all. No emotional entanglements, no hours of plotting and planning, no pissed-off lovers. Gavin wouldn't have to know. At least not right away. After all, I never told him when I booked with Ricky. Was there really a big difference?

By the time the taxi crossed the invisible Bronx border, I was committed. *Why not?* I asked myself. *I'm due. No. I'm overdue.*

When I got out of the cab and paid the driver, my mind was already churning over the next steps. All I needed was some good, solid research to find my man hands. I'd just taken my first step through the looking glass.

Chapter Four

Outside My Box

THAT NIGHT, THE boys were in their room with the door closed and Gavin was snoring on the couch. Boys. I use that term loosely. My sons were closer to being men. The younger, Ben, had patches of peach fuzz, and Andrew suddenly sported a perpetual five o'clock shadow. Ben was undoubtedly lost to *World of Warcraft,* his infuriating computer-game addiction. Andrew was probably talking to his girlfriend, running up the cell-phone bill.

Last but not least, Gavin. He was clearly more intrigued by professional billiards on TV than talking. I looked over at his familiar form—balding head, red beard, and spreading paunch—planted in front of the TV and saw him slump over his laptop. I marveled that anyone could pass out in that position. I poked him. He keeled over onto his side. Same thing every night.

"Gavin. Go to bed."

He grunted and, seemingly still asleep, made his way into the bedroom area while telepathically avoiding sneakers, DVD cases, and balled-up clothes. I went barefoot, picking up all manner of junk, bussing crusty dishes, sweeping up crumbs and bits of unidentifiable matter. I had to do it, otherwise I couldn't function. It's not like I was a neat freak, but with limited space—which included my home-office hideaway desk and four outsized personalities—it was up to me to make room. It had become my evening custom. I wrestled a small plastic shopping bag of trash into the building's communal garbage chute and let fly a string of curses that would give Bitsy a run for her money. I was impatient. I had a date with a computer winking an invitation into an exotic world. I needed to get to it, now.

With the apartment far from spotless, I settled into my velveteen recliner, propped myself up with pillows, and arranged my aging Dell and a glass of full-bodied burgundy on the portable desk tray. The quiet and the cool breeze that swept through the room cleared my head. I loosened my fingers and got ready to launch the world's sexiest search. *Women, Massage, Sensual,* I typed into Google. The computer wheezed and cranked, and finally coughed up page after page of possibilities. For men. Straight or gay, it didn't matter. If men wanted touch, they could get touch. What a selection. Dominatrices, horny college girls, lonely Russian housewives, Asian princesses—"Direct Descendants of Genghis Kahn!"—and women who specialized in huge breasts and even bigger butts. It's a wonder that we have only one or two government scandals a month.

For women, it was as dry as the desert. I followed one hyperlink after another and got nothing. Was it possible that I was the only woman who desired sexual touch? I quickly dismissed the idea—if my job had taught me one thing, it was that you're never the only one. There were plenty of infertile couples twenty years ago, only no one talked about it.

The longer I trawled, the angrier and more frustrated I got. There was nothing equal opportunity about this. Why couldn't I have a sensual massage? Why was this for men only? It was almost 1:30. I decided to give it one more shot before I threw in the towel.

After a fruitless week, I switched search engines. They don't call it "Yahoo!" for nothing. SoHo Touch in NYC came right up. The home page was a tasteful, arty photo of the curve of a naked hip, the name in an elegant font. I almost mistook it for a design studio until I looked closer. "Sensual massage for men and women." Women! I couldn't believe my eyes. I read the entire site about a dozen times. SoHo Touch offered organic Lotus Touch massage cream and special music that made the brain produce pleasure-enhancing alpha and theta waves. I had no idea! And yet it sounded like any other spa, except for the few special services on the menu. I clicked on a panoramic view of the spa—an expansive, bright, exclusive space. It looked like the promised land.

I woke up too early the next morning, downed too many cups of coffee, and gave my boys the bum's rush out the door. I needed to compose myself so I could make the SoHo Touch connection. I was grateful for the morning solitude, that small window after the guys left and before the cascade of business calls. It was a treasured perk of working at home. My virtual office connected me to my far-flung employees, all of us computer commuters.

I dialed. My hands shook, my stomach backflipped. This was so naughty. So scary. I almost hung up when a woman picked up.

"SoHo Touch. How may I help you?"

"Is it true? Do you offer sensual massage to women?" My mouth was so dry the words stuck to my tongue.

"Oh yes, all the time." Her matter-of-factness was reassuring. "Do you want a woman?"

"Oh no! No. Nooo . . . " She'd caught me off guard. "Don't you have men who massage women?"

"Yes, we can have a man for you," she offered.

"When is your next available appointment?" Did I just say that? What I really wanted to know was who was he, what did he look like, can I see a picture, what's he going to do to me, what do I wear, do a lot of women do this? I must have telegraphed anxiety. She was on it.

"You can rest assured that SoHo Touch has been assisting women for a very long time," she said in a dulcet, pseudo-British accent. "Our policy requires a hostess to greet you at the door and remain in the space at all times. Next Tuesday is open if it fits with your schedule."

She made it seem ordinary. I wasn't the only one. What a relief. Moreover, there was a full-fledged service for plucky female explorers like me.

"May I have your name, please?"

"My name? Um, Kate. Kate's my name." I gave the first one that came into my head. *The Taming of the Shrew.* I always loved that play.

"Someone will call you in a few days to let you know the address, Kate. The fee is $300 for a two-hour session. SoHo Touch accepts cash and all major credit cards." I gulped at the tag. Pricey. But really, I rationalized, not all that much more than a good eucalyptus scrub and a hot rock massage. "Okay, then, good. I'll be there Tuesday."

Before I could change my mind, I hung up. I steadied the jitters with a bagel and cheese, my equivalent of a scotch on the rocks. The second thing I did was call Beth. After a lifetime of being the first to know all my secret confidences—dates, blow jobs, sex, my first (and only) clandestine joyride with boys, proposal, engagement, pregnancies, and betrayals—she'd kill me if I didn't tell her before anyone else. That would be cheating on her.

"Guess what I am doing?" Without waiting for a response, I told her.

"Are you crazy? Have you lost all your marbles? Jeez! You're not serious, are you?" Beth was beside herself. This was the first out-of-character, risky, sexy thing that I'd ever done in my life. She clearly wasn't ready for it.

"What do you know about this place? Who are these people? You could be walking into a den of murderers or white-slave traders. Have you thought about that?"

"Actually, Beth, I've always wanted to be abducted. I'm sure I'm exactly what a sultan would pay big bucks for: a slightly used, zaftig, loud Jewess. Of course I've thought about it, you moron. It's why I'm giving you the name, the address, the phone number, and a place to wait for me. I know you want to be there. I'm arranging a par-tay. Everybody who's anybody will be there. Olivia, Vicki, Sophia. My posse of pussy protectors. If I'm not out by 5:15, storm the castle."

"You're such a show-off. Wouldn't it be easier to have a quiet, simple affair like everyone else?"

"Not from what I've seen watching you ladies. I couldn't handle the drama. All that 'torn between two lovers' stuff. It would make me schizy. All the secret phone calls and hot-sheet rendezvous while trying to work out the marriage kinks in couples therapy. It would be too much for my little brain. And you know how shitty I am at keeping a secret. That doesn't mean I don't want *something.* This could be the something."

"Touché!" After a beat she asked, "In that case, Snow White, are you telling Gavin?"

I took a breath. "No. Not yet. This is merely a massage, with sensual overtones, organic Lotus Touch massage cream, and theta brain waves. What's to tell?"

Beth stifled a gag. "Blech."

"Thanks for your support, kiddo. Enough about me. You hanging in there? How're the girls? Have things settled down between you and Kevin?"

"Well, it's easier with Larry working late every night. But it's insane that Kev's jealous whenever I get along with my husband. I can never talk about Larry with Kev on any level. It upsets him too much. I don't know, maybe I should just break it off with him. . . . He needs too much attention."

This wasn't the first time that Kev's neediness had pushed Beth to the wall. But I knew he touched something inside her that she needed. I didn't think she could end things with him. At least, not now. I held my tongue and followed our default agreement: Whenever the men in our lives were giving us trouble, we'd just say, "He's a great big hairy asshole."

"Oh, Beth, Kev can be a great big hairy asshole sometimes."

"Thank you. That was the perfect thing to say," Beth said, letting a little light into her heavy mood. "Go call the rest of the Martini Gang. I know you're dying to tell them. I gotta drop off the girls anyway. I swear, sometimes I'm just running a taxi service."

"Okay. I'll check on you later."

I got right back on the phone and called my posse. With only minor variations, each one thought I'd lost it. *Au contraire.* I thought that, just maybe, I'd finally found it.

Chapter Five

Move Over, Pussy Galore

I WAS ON PINS and needles. Next Tuesday seemed years away. I compensated the only way I knew how—I threw myself into hyperdrive. I took the kids to get new sneakers. Ben needed his braces tightened. Andrew, a recent vegetarian convert, gave me a shopping list of organic greens. I made the rounds of the New York City reproductive doctors squeezing out their yearly pledges to underwrite patient education. I stopped at every hot dog and pretzel stand along the way.

I did a pretty good job of putting SoHo Touch on my brain's back burner until the alarm went off Tuesday morning. I jumped out of bed. Omigod. SoHo Touch. I was going for the most expensive rubdown I'd ever had. I was going to get man hands.

I didn't know how to calm myself. I couldn't eat one more thing. I meditated on Samantha Jones, the most sexually honest woman I've ever encountered, even if she wasn't real. *Sex and the City* was my only blueprint for becoming an adventurous woman. I was considerably shorter, darker, and fatter than Ms. Jones, but I could still be daring, sophisticated, and sexy. At least, I told myself I could.

At eleven a.m., the phone call came. A seductive male voice with Clive Owen plumminess revealed the ultrasecret, überhip downtown Manhattan location. "Once inside the building, Kate, look for the door with the red ribbon."

Behind the door, he promised a well-appointed loft with a stocked bar and food. "Do try to be exactly on time," he instructed. "Do not come early." The cloak-and-dagger aspect of it ratcheted up my anticipation, which was already at nosebleed levels.

Three o'clock was an eternity away. I couldn't figure out what to do with myself for four whole hours. I puttered aimlessly for a few minutes, made a couple of work calls—none of which I could remember. I filled the tub with warm water scented with lavender salts and eased myself into the aromatic brew. I wanted to soak myself into a sensuous mood, but the minute I looked down at my abundant body, with its rolling hills and valleys, I felt defeated. I wasn't a sleek downtown type. I couldn't remember the last time I got a catcall or even a glance from a construction worker. The hot woman in me was buried under the same sixty pounds I'd needed to lose ever since Ben was born. I'd managed to make myself sexually invisible. I couldn't imagine any man wanting to touch this, even if I paid him. I hated my body. I was sick of being "the girl with the pretty face."

As I lay there, dripping wet and bummed, my big sexual exploit seemed like the dumbest idea ever. But this was my cliff and damn it, I was jumping off even if I was terrified. Pity the poor man who was assigned to give me a sensual massage. He was going to have his hands full.

I dried off and lathered on expensive creams. At least I could smell good for the guy. I chose my outfit as if clothes mattered. I found my New York City chic-yet-artsy uniform: black pants, black sweater, and jacket. Best of all, it hid my ass. I was leaving comfortably middle-class, middle-of-the-road Riverdale for SoHo, the land of skinny, well-heeled hipsters. One does want to blend in, doesn't one?

I drove down Manhattan's West Side to the southern end of the island. I had ample time to nibble a light lunch and sip a very dirty martini to loosen myself up.

With another forty-five minutes to kill, I walked over to Babeland, a women-friendly sex-toy store a couple of blocks away. How thoughtful of Big Brother—I mean, Yahoo!—to advertise Babeland right on my e-mail page. Touring the shop was like visiting an alternate universe. The "toys" weren't anything I'd ever played with. They were laid out with the kind of care usually reserved for the Barneys designer shoe department. With slightly amused, sympathetic smiles, the attentive all-girl staff watched me gawk. I had a lot of questions and, with a few ounces of vodka lubricating my tongue, I let 'em rip.

"Exactly how does this work?" I asked, holding up a fleshy-feeling contraption with protuberances all over. A sweet-faced girl in a kilt, biker boots, and heavy wrist cuffs gave me a seriously X-rated explanation, lisping around her tongue piercings. Halfway through her no-blush-no-fuss spiel, I spaced out. I was having trouble following the anatomy lesson that was essential if you were going to propel yourself into orgasmic orbit with this gizmo. "I'll take it," I said. I left with a pink Rabbit.

At 2:55 p.m., I found the top-secret building. By 2:58, I was in front of the ribbon-festooned door.

I checked my watch, willing the minute hand to move to twelve. By 2:59, my resolve was just about gone and my heartbeat was arrhythmic. I concentrated on the Martini Gang, stationed at a nearby bar waiting on high alert until they got my all clear. They knew where to find me.

It was a little Ian Flemingish, but I needed my girls at my back. I checked my watch, again. Three o'clock. I steadied one hand with the other and rang the buzzer. The door opened before I had a chance to flee. A twentysomething woman—tall, lanky, and brunette—graciously welcomed me by name.

"Kate, we have been expecting you." Her voice was velvet. "I'm Angelique." She was so downtown cool, I immediately tripped on the doorsill.

I don't know what I expected, but it certainly wasn't this nonchalance. I did love hearing myself called Kate. I'd practiced "Kate" in my head every day since I booked the appointment. My new *nom de sex* added to my bad-girl persona. I felt I'd been liberated from my Pamela self. Almost.

The loft was an *Architectural Digest* masterpiece, decorated with sleek sofas, lots of easy chairs, and a big-screen TV. The hostess showed me to the bar, where a guy in his midthirties hunched over a bowl of peanuts. He was stocky with a shaved head, kind of bland. Since he was the only man there, except for the bartender, I deduced he must be my guy. When the hostess introduced me to Boris, I fought the disappointment. I was hoping for someone prettier, with a more chiseled face, maybe dressed in a fireman's outfit. I smiled at the thought. I didn't know what I wanted, not really. But when I saw him, I knew he wasn't it.

Breathe, I silently repeated like a mantra. *In and out, in and out, that's all you have to do.* My heart was going like a souped-up Ferrari when, for some inexplicable reason, my husband popped into my head. Not in a million years, not in his wildest imagination would he ever picture me here. The thought of the look on his face if he knew provoked uncontrollable laughter. Boris shifted uncomfortably in his seat. I tried to stifle the next wave of hooting. "I'm sorry, I'm just nervous," I apologized.

The hostess retreated with a polite little bow. This was the real thing. I wanted to throw up. Instead, I smiled awkwardly. Boris, looking slightly bored, led me to a back area where there were five massage rooms.

"Here ve are." His heavy Eastern European accent made me work to understand him. He ushered me into a sparse room: a table, a place for my clothes, and that was it. He put out a bathrobe and told me he was going to run a shower for me across the hall. "After shower, ve vill begin. I vait for you."

Shower? All those lovely creams. I was a freaking flower! What a waste. I grabbed the overlaundered, no-longer-white robe, jammed my feet into the plastic flip-flops, and made my way across the hall.

I dodged under the water, rinsed off quickly, wrapped the robe tightly around myself, and scurried back to the room. Looking at the massage table and Boris gave me a bad case of the shakes. I was wet, cold, and rattled by doubt. *Do you really want to do this? Now? Ever?* I steeled myself and asked my "therapist" if we could talk for a minute before beginning.

"Look," I said, "I have never done this before. I am a married woman. Married for more than twenty years. I have never, ever been touched in a sexual way by anyone beside my husband. So, could you please go slowly? I'm really a very nice girl."

Boris looked at me like I had just landed from Planet What-the-Hell-Are-You-Talking-About. He grunted, "Ah huh."

We stood in dead silence, locked in a weird stare-down for what felt like forever before he blurted, "Take off de robe and ged on de table."

With that, he departed. I looked around for something to cover me—a sheet, a towel, a Kleenex. There was nothing. I stuck my head out of the room. "Excuse me? I need a cover sheet!"

Boris was bewildered by the request. "Cover sheet?" He came

back into the room, rummaged in a couple of drawers, and pulled out a towel. Clearly, I was missing the point of this whole exercise if I wanted a cover. Sensual massage implied nudity. I was overcome by a modesty that made me feel clumsy and embarrassed. This was not the erotic me I had envisioned. "Once I become more relaxed maybe we can see about removing it," I said, and continued to chatter a mile a minute, making excuses as if I weren't paying for the privilege of having Boris work on me.

"Ah huh." Boris was one smooth dude. I got on the table. He wanted me on my stomach, which, thankfully, felt right—safer, more familiar, like a regular massage. I put my face in the cradle with the towel over my backside, closed my eyes, and tried to settle down.

With the niceties out of the way, Boris began. He dumped warm oil over every millimeter of my exposed body until I was one giant oil slick. With his big, heavy hands, he started to work my flesh. With every move, he sent me sliding from one side of the table to the other. I held on for dear life. It didn't take long for me to get into it, though. Oohhh. Mmm. Good pressure. Long strokes. This was it? What's the big deal? I could do this. My breathing slowed and I let myself feel wanton, a sex goddess on training wheels. Take that, Beth! Olivia! Vicki! Sophia! And yeah, you too, Ricky!

I was doing fine—even feeling a little cocky—when Boris shoved each of my legs to either side of the table. There I was, splayed like a frog for dissection, the towel slipping. Ricky didn't do that at the spa. Boris moved up and down my back into territory not previously traveled. Hands were going in and out of my inner thighs, around my bottom. My breath quickened. This must be the sensual part. Not only could I do this, I could like this. With Angelique, the velvet hostess stationed outside my door, fluffing pillows and offering a gin and tonic to some other eager client, I could relax and have fun. Then, for no explainable reason, Boris switched up his stoke. He began hammering, chop-chopping with enthusiastic effort like a trainer working on his boxer. Me, I'm not into blood sport. It was impossible to feel sexy, let alone unwind, while Boris tenderized me like a chicken cutlet.

It went on forever until Boris asked me to turn over. The moment of truth. The towel was completely missing and I'd be damned if I was going to ask for it back. I sucked air and flipped around, skidding perilously close to the edge. In what was apparently his trademark maneuver, he pinned my legs to the sides of the table. More oil. He ran his hands in smooth, long strokes over my torso. I was braced for the chop, but it didn't come. After a couple of minutes, I softened . . . mmm . . . I did like this. *I am a repressed but shameless hedonist,* I thought. *One right move and I become a puddle of surrender.* Boris checked in. "You are alr-r-r-ight? Fe-e-els gut?"

"Um-hmm," I sighed as he roamed the landscape of my breasts and down my belly to my inner thighs. He was careful to avoid the vulva, but it was suggestive enough. Just as I was heating up, I felt the blows. Boris, now forever known as the Chopster, was an amateur.

"Have you worked on many women?" I asked in my most gentle, nonjudgmental way. I didn't want to rile him while he was flailing away at my naked self.

"No," he admitted. "But I straight. Mostly, I verk on de gay boys at a place in downtown. I like de girls! Not de boys!"

Party over. "Thank you," I told him between blows. "Thank you so much. But I am feeling like I have had enough lovely touch."

Boris grunted a response before leaving me. I slid off the oil-drenched table and skidded back to the shower to clean up the environmental disaster that was my body. I got dressed in a hurry, then rendezvoused with Boris at the bar. His face creased in concern as I pressed a wad of bills into his hands. "I vas gut? You enchoy your-r-r-self?" He sounded so worried, I had no choice but to lie.

"You were wonderful," I told him, staring directly into his eyes. I can be so convincing when I want to be.

"Vy?" he wanted to know. "Vy you are payink for dis massage? You are wery pretty. You vould not haf to pay for a man to touch you. Many mens vould enchoy touchink you."

Good question, Chopster, why *was* I doing this? I tried to explain that I didn't want to make problems in my marriage.

"I don't want the complications of an affair. I don't want to actually have sex," I concluded. "I just want to have a sensual experience in a way that isn't going to hurt anybody. Like men get to do."

With that I gathered up my pride and checked myself in the mirror on the way out. Right behind me, too close for comfort, was another client. A man. We were practically back-to-belly in the cramped hallway waiting for the elevator, until he couldn't take one more second and ran for the stairs.

On the solo ride down, I punched in Beth's cell number before I even made it to the street.

"I'm alive!" I announced when she picked up.

Squeals from the other end of the line. "Omigod. Sweetie! How are you? How was, um, it? C'mon, we're dyin' here." I could hear her switch to the tinny speakerphone.

I told the gang the truth. "Parts of it were exciting and other parts were so-so. Some were just bizarre."

I speed-walked to meet them for the drinks I had promised. When I got to the restaurant they examined me closely for signs of . . . something.

"Was it an adventure?"

"Oh, yes. Yes it was."

"Are you going to go back?"

"No way," I yelped like I'd been goosed. Calmly, I conceded, "I gotta confess, plotting it, picturing it was way better than the actual thing. The guy was incompetent. Nice enough and totally safe. But he had no idea what he was doing."

"So are you going to give up on this cockamamy idea, Mrs. Gay Man?" Vicki said. "What about JDate? Someone just told me about a site totally devoted to cheating spouses. There are so many other options that don't cost a cent. What about it?"

"Give up? Why would I do that? There were moments that were actually good. I just haven't found the right man hands yet. I deserve this. And I still think there's a way of getting what I need without having an affair. I know there's more to sensual massage than a barrel of sweet crude and a light bruising. I can make this work."

Without quite meaning to, I had found my new mission.

Chapter Six

Birth of an Everyday Supergoddess, or, First You Ask Your Son

There had to be one professional sexy-touch masseur in New York City who was competent with women. My bar wasn't that high. There's no insult intended here, but I had been eating the same entrée for over twenty years—it was tasty, but predictable. I kept fantasizing about a five-star tasting menu full of new flavors. I made up my mind that I was going to sample them with the same clean pay-for-play that any man, straight or gay, could have. I just needed some direction.

"Ricky, spill it," I dug in the minute he picked up his private line. "Where do you find these guys?"

"I'm fine, thanks, Pam. What are you talking about?"

"I want to know how you find these masseurs who make you purr and then send you back to your hubby. I want one of those. Now."

"Omigod, Pamela. What have I unleashed?" His nervous giggles filled the line. "Gavin is going to kill me. Your mother is going to kill me."

For a split second, I went there. If Gavin was going to kill anyone, it was going to be me. Not that Gavin was capable of murder. He was a gentle man. Of course I had guilt about having desires that didn't include my husband. But I had just gotten a taste of sensuality that was strictly about me, and it was electrifying. Even though Boris was an overall letdown, he had given me a glimpse of what was possible. When his hands rolled over my breasts, I was taken out of my head, out of my obsessive worry that my body was too imperfect to ever be beautiful. Despite the oil slick and karate chops, Boris made me feel desirable. The idea of feeling sexual without having to think about satisfying my husband was extraordinarily liberating. If there were risks, I was willing to take them to feel that again for more than a minute. And the pursuit of it, the cloak-and-dagger setup, had certainly been a thrill. I was starting to enjoy feeling a little reckless.

"Shut up, Ricky. Give me a name."

Another peal of anxious laughter. "All right, all right. I go to MassageM4M.com. How that's going to help you, I don't know. But that's where I go."

Before he could say another word, I hung up and started mapping my expedition into gay-man's-land.

The dishes were in the washer. I was finishing up a call with Bob, one of my organization's more involved board members. We'd just saved the monthly newsletter from being hijacked by a Midwestern printer who figured he could boost his price two days before deadline. With the exquisite precision of a practiced good cop–bad cop team, Bob and I beat him back. Bob wanted to savor the victory. I wanted to get the hell off the phone. Usually I liked schmoozing with him. At this moment, he was a roadblock on my way to M4M.

"Bob, I don't know about you, but I'm whipped." With the humid summer night draining what was left of my energy, I considered telling him what I was up to. It'd be so much easier. We were well on the way to becoming best buds, checking in every day, talking about everything under the sun except work. He was another gay man who couldn't get enough sex talk. In fact, he was starved for it. Texas wasn't the most gay-friendly state. I had recruited Bob to serve on the board, and my instincts about him were paying off. He was a lot of fun, a great blend of business acumen, quick wit, and sympathetic insights—an ideal addition. I started to say something but stopped myself. I had to fight my impulse to invite him into my life the way I always did when I liked someone. That intimate informality was my trademark, or my pathology, depending on your perspective. It created a culture that was warm and supportive and made the organization successful. But we weren't close enough for me to smuggle him over the border into my personal life. I zipped my lips, blew him a kiss good-bye, and hung up.

Finally I could give my laptop my full attention. I smacked the keys to get a flicker on the dark screen.

"You're gonna break it, Pam," Gavin grumbled from the sofa, sixty percent TV-narcotized, forty percent asleep. How'd he do that? I called his name fifteen times a day, and he didn't answer. The minute he got a hint of bad behavior around electronics, his antennae were up and waving.

The old Dell made promising noises. "Sorry, honey. Go back to sleep."

I watched Gavin drop back into sleep. The screen blinked to life, and what a life it was. Men. Nothing but men. Muscled men. Slender men. Manly men. Glittery men with unnaturally long eyelashes. Some guys advertised themselves with professional headshots, while others featured only extreme close-ups of apparently pertinent body parts.

They all shared the promise of sensual massage. I weeded out the ones who seemed to promise a whole lot more. I concentrated on the language, not the photos, although I have to say those were riveting. Five or six ads used the same terms: "Body Electric," "Sacred Intimacy," and something called "power, surrender, and intimacy." This was all new to me, but those words implied something deeper than a quick fix for an erotic emergency.

I couldn't stop reading. These sensual or erotic massage services were deeply rooted in gay culture, a lot of it born as a safe-sex response to the AIDS crisis. I respected that. But clearly, as a girl, I was going to have to get creative.

What if I wrote to these guys? What if I asked if they'd be willing to work on female anatomy? I'd either be giving them a good laugh or a whole new market. I was an entrepreneurial opportunity. All I needed was the guts to do it. What's the worst that could happen?

My own three guys were out cold on the couch looking like a mountain of unfolded laundry. I couldn't help noticing that I didn't feel a twinge of remorse. I loved them and I was happy they were there. I also was delighted that they were unconscious.

I scrolled through the pages before I found one masseur who wasn't promoting his hard hoo-ha. He didn't even have a picture, just vaguely Hallmark-y text about the healing power of touch and inner experiences. Healing sounded good to me and not at all threatening.

I was about to write to him when lightning struck. The minute I hit the Send key I'd be out there, exposed. Cyber-naked. I may be a techno idiot, but I knew enough to know that whatever pseudonym I used, if I sent an e-mail from my regular e-mail address, I could be tracked down faster than a circus elephant on a rampage in midtown Manhattan. Everybody in my family and the organization I worked for was on the same general account. That's all I needed, one private e-mail straying into the professional bin and buh-bye career. It'd be all over the fertility field in the time it took to hit Forward. And what if my kids got curious?

There was only one answer: a secret e-mail account. I had no idea how to set one up. Gavin was my guru and I wasn't quite ready for that husband-and-wife sit-down. I did the next best thing. I asked my son.

"Sweetheart. Andrew. Honey. Wake up." I gently shook him. "Could you please help me with the computer?"

Andrew rubbed the sleep from his eyes. I made my request, and he shot me his patented quizzical-with-irony look. "What are you up to, Mom?" His face crinkled in a wry smile that made me extremely uncomfortable.

"Look, Andrew, Mom just needs some privacy, okay? Don't you ever like to post on boards and don't want people to know it's you?" Guilt coated every word and raised my voice an octave. The kid peered at me like I was committing a felony. My cheeks burned.

"Sure, Mom. Whatever you say." He didn't buy any of it, but he showed me how to set up the account.

"Okay. Now, what name do you want?" Bang. Blindsided by the obvious question. Let the blustering commence.

"Yes, Mom. Name. That was the whole point. What's your new e-mail handle?" Andrew inherited his father's penchant for logic.

"Honey, that's Mommy's business," I said. Did I say "Mommy"? He hasn't called me "Mommy" in eleven years. "I haven't quite decided yet. Anyway, I can take it from here."

"Are you sure?"

"Yes, Mommy is sure. Now go!" I was talking about myself in the third person. Never a good sign.

"Yeah, okay, Mom-mee. Whatever makes you happy." Andrew turned to leave the office portion of the living room for the TV-viewing section, but then he looked over his shoulder and winked conspiratorially. "Have fun and don't do anything I wouldn't do."

The sarcasm was definitely from my side of the family. I watched him settle back on the couch next to Gavin and Ben and slip the remote out of his snoring dad's hand.

Alone at last, figuratively speaking. I cranked up the air conditioner and sat with my fingers poised over the keyboard. A name. What's in a name? Everything. All of a sudden I was having an identity crisis. I was ready to become someone else. But who? I knew my name would have to project the essential but unseen me—sultry, juicy, a little mysterious, unattainable, and the opposite of the everyday, accessible, can-do caregiver Pam.

With Liz Phair singing in my earbuds about being a sexy, psycho supergoddess, I fished for ideas. I put the new terms I discovered on M4M into my search engine and the floodgates opened. Suddenly, it was all Tantra, all the time. On the new sites that popped up, the men were replaced by "goddesses" of the sensual realm. Goddess Aloha bathed men in special rituals; Goddess Jasmine gave guys sacred-spot massage lessons, whatever those were; Goddess Shirley taught men how to cultivate sexual energy with hands-on techniques that "left no part untouched." If only I had testicles, I could "relax deeply on the Altar of the Light Body in the candlelit Transformation Center" as three or four bindi-wearing goddesses, who were about as Indian as my mother, brought me to a place of deep pleasure.

There was not a horny Russian housewife or naughty schoolgirl in the pantheon. Anyone and everyone in the Tantra universe was a practitioner of the "sacred erotic arts." They got tributes, not tips. They worked in temples, not brothels. Theirs was a higher calling.

The New Age spiritual approach to sex was feeling pretty good. Quite wholesome, actually. I could relate. I could be a goddess. I didn't know how, but I could start by calling myself one.

HidingGoddess@I'm-not-gonna-tell-you.com was born.

Finding one's identity is so fatiguing. I fell asleep in my chair.

Chapter Seven

If I Was a Gay Man, Ya Ha Deedle Deedle, Bubba Bubba Deedle Deedle Dum

I WAS PUMPED AND prepared the next night when I visited M4M. I knew my odds of getting a response were low, but so what? It was worth a shot. All I needed was one out of the hundreds of sensual masseurs to take me, ovaries and all. So many of them were absolutely beautiful. It was like perusing a case of artisanal Boston cream pies, walnut coffee rings, and buttercream layer cakes. Surely there was bound to be one risk-taking capitalist cupcake among them.

I ended up writing to five men who focused on "Body Electric" and "Tantra," and the "sacred" sexual experience. They conscientiously avoided any X-rated suggestions, and by now, I had decoded the terms well enough to figure out that they weren't offering sleazy quickies. Their posts had a spiritual ring, promising enlightenment through sexuality. Enlightenment. Perfect. I was so done with living in the dark.

With all the pieces in place, I made my first foray.

I know that you are a gay man, but would you consider working on a woman? I don't want anything more than sensual massage. What do you think?

Sincerely yours,

Hiding Goddess

I hit Send with a finger full of swagger. Within a few hours, Sam popped up:

Dear Hiding Goddess,

I have never worked on a woman before, but I am open to expanding my practice. Where can I reach you so that we can connect by phone?

I read it over obsessively. Sam seemed genuine enough. At least there were no overt signs of borderline personality disorder. "Girl, you are so fucking crazy," I said to myself in tender encouragement as I responded with my mobile number. *Call anytime over the weekend.*

The days went by in a blur of business meetings. The monthly newsletter was short two articles. That's what you get when you ask people to write for free. In a panic, I put a badgering phone call in to Bitsy. She grudgingly yielded, offering a reworked version of an article she'd just published in a journal on the legal complications of surrogacy and egg donation.

"Bits, you're the best. Can you get this done by tomorrow?"

"Absolutely not! Tomorrow's Saturday. I can't. I have errands to run. And a date tonight."

I couldn't believe she'd tried to slip that by me.

"A date? That's so great! Who? Is he cute? You mean eHarmony works? What's he do?"

Bitsy's silence was loaded. She wasn't going to tell me, or anyone, the details until after the fact. But she relented on the article. "Okay, okay. I'll get up early and you'll have it by noon."

I was looking forward to hearing about her adventure in date world. Maybe this would take her edge off. Or blunt it a little.

I woke up early the next morning and piled the trunk and backseat of the car with fresh meats, corn, and salad fixings for our Long Island beach house BBQ later that evening. My eightysomething mother walked briskly over from her apartment just a few blocks away and installed herself in the passenger seat. We hit the road and bumper-to-bumper traffic.

I was dreading that Sam would choose this moment to call. I couldn't have this conversation in front of my mother. My mother, with her seer's gift for knowing things, wouldn't give it a rest if she overheard me scheduling. She'd be even more suspicious if I didn't answer a call. I always talked in front of her. Roz knew everything about my friends—the dramas, the infidelities, the sorrow. She never judged them. Only me. Mercifully, the only person who called was Bitsy, with a report on the "schmuck" of a date and to tell me that the article was done.

Gavin met us at the dock in the flat-bottom motorboat we used to ferry things and people to our beach house on the small island a mere few hundred feet from the mainland.

"My parents are here," he said, loading up the last of the food and helping my mother into the boat. "They docked their houseboat late last night. They look great."

"I don't know how they live on that ship," Roz volunteered. "The bathroom is so small."

"Head, Roz. It's called the head," Gavin instructed.

"Head, schmead. It's too small."

We shared the summer bungalow with Gavin's brother, his wife, and their kids. With my in-laws, my mother, and my two boys, plus Andrew's girlfriend visiting, the tiny house was throbbing. I was wound so tight that I didn't have my usual patience for our family's chitchat. I jumped out of my skin when my mobile went off.

"I need to answer this," I announced.

"For crissakes, Pammy, you have to work the one freaking weekend we're all out here?" Gavin was pissed, and the top of his sunburned head turned redder—would it kill him to wear a hat?

Mostly, he really was good about the constant disruptions and intrusions. He accepted that helping infertile people was my mission. After we got clobbered with infertility, I gave up my gig as a kindergarten teacher and devoted myself to the unpaid glories of patient advocacy. Gavin was 100 percent behind my newfound activism. The emotional and financial beatings we took trying to have children had brought him onto my bandwagon. Every now and then, though, the relentlessness of it got to him and he'd erupt in a "your job or me" rage.

"Go. But hurry up," he snapped. I left him muttering under his breath and hustled off the wooden porch and down the sandy path along the shore to return Sam's call in private.

Sam was polite, a little nervous-sounding, and not nearly as slick as the SoHo Touch front desk. In fact, the first thing he did was give me kudos for having the courage to e-mail him.

"I understand how hard it can be to reach out of your comfort zone for something you need, Kate."

"Thank you. I can't tell you how much better it makes me feel hearing you say that," I said. "I'm really new at this. Frankly, my first and only time trying sensual massage wasn't exactly a home run."

"Well, as I said in my note, Kate, I don't have any experience working with women. But I have years of working with men who are trying to heal life issues through touch and their bodies. I don't imagine it's that different for you. I'm happy to try to help you, too."

His honesty and earnestness embarrassed me almost as much

as it relieved me. Sam was a true therapist willing to work with me on my terms and I hadn't even given him my real name.

"Sam, you sound like a lovely person. And I want to be honest with you, too. The way you talk makes me feel safe enough to tell you my name's not Kate, it's Pam."

He laughed. "Thank you for trusting me, Pam. Now, how can I help you? What are you looking for? You might not know this, but I have years of working with urologists to help their patients with erectile dysfunction, premature ejaculation, and prostate cancer. Important issues."

Great news—if I had a dick. On the other hand, compared to Boris, Sam was a gentleman poet. I accepted his limitations as a fact of life. He was gay, after all. Sure, I hoped that he'd had a girlfriend or two before he figured it out. But you take what you can get.

I confessed that I didn't know what I wanted, other than that I longed to connect with my own sensuality. I also confessed to wanting to feel that from someone other than my husband. Not that I wanted to sacrifice my marriage. That was the whole point of paying for professional massage therapy—it didn't break my marriage vows, and maybe it could bring me into a sensual space that Gavin didn't need to be a part of.

I made a tentative appointment for the following Tuesday and hurried back along the sand to the house. Gavin was ticked. He flipped steaks on the grill so hard they almost bounced off. "So, Pam, did you blaze new trails, make the world a safer place for the reproductively challenged?"

"Yes, darling," I answered sweetly, grabbing the BBQ tongs from his fist. "I absolutely did."

Even though experts recommend having dinner together every night, my typical American family couldn't pull that off except on these rare occasions during the summer. The kids sat at one end of the gigantic picnic table shouting incomprehensible teen shorthand at each other, laughing hysterically, while my father-in-law openly ogled Andrew's practically naked eighteen-year-old girlfriend.

"Could that bathing suit get any smaller?" my mother whispered loud enough for the next-door neighbors to hear. She poked me in the ribs and nodded toward Ben. "Don't you underestimate your youngest. Ben is a looker and he's going to be very successful. I predict it."

"He'll be the next Warren Buffett if he remembers to do his homework."

As soon as the sun sank low enough, the bugs came out with a furious hunger. We fled inside. My God, it was a small house. As the first pellets of rain hit the roof, my claustrophobia erupted. It was impossible to sleep. I couldn't wait until daylight to get off the island. By 8 a.m., I was packed and ready. The kids stayed behind and Gavin, still ticked at me, went to the office.

"At least I'll have some peace. No one will be there on Sunday."

It was official. I was in the doghouse. I'd deal with it later. By 8:30, I was driving back to Riverdale with my mother riding shotgun, her mouth on automatic.

"Pammy, I was thinking how you're one step away from being your old self again. So beautiful. That's why you should take off the weight before menopause. Because after, the skin gets loose. It just doesn't snap back like when you're younger."

I shot her a look, trying not to give in to the fleeting but intense loathing only daughters can have for their mothers, or to let the usual self-hating reaction take hold. I coped in silence and pushed the speed limit the whole way home, pulling up in front of her building and nearly shoving her out of the car. "I'll call you soon," I promised.

Seven minutes later, I locked myself into my apartment with my new obsession. I had all 800 square feet to myself. I cranked up the computer, plunked myself at the table, and went right for Sam's Web site, searching for a picture. There he was on the About page, an unremarkable, fortyish man with a full beard and soulful eyes. His soft gaze did nothing for me.

On the other hand, I did like the way Sam wrote passionately and elegantly about the power of erotic touch. It was the first time I had heard a man speak about the deeper possibilities. *Erotic touch is a pathway to bridging the disconnect that so many of us suffer when we can't unite heart, mind, and body. This ancient practice, with its roots in Tantra and Kundalini yoga, is designed to bring each client into wholeness.*

Like everybody else I knew, I was searching for one integrated self. Sam struck a resonating chord with me: I was a woman in pieces, when I wanted to be a woman at peace. Most of us women play a bunch of disjointed roles in life. It's exhausting. I'd spent years in a therapist's office trying to sort it out. I'd absorbed a little of the yoga sutras, Zen Buddhism, and the teachings of countless self-help gurus to learn the trick of knitting together my disparate elements. No matter what I tried, though, I remained daughter, sister, wife, mother, executive director, advocate, spokesperson, and best girlfriend. When I wasn't one thing, I had to be the other. It was as if I didn't exist outside of those roles. Sitting alone in silence was unbearable. I was frightened of myself, plagued by anxiety that I was too big in every possible way. In a lifelong war with my own body, I hated my weight and my inability to shed those last demoralizing inches. Yes, all of this was wrapped up in an outwardly successful package: a happy wife, mother, sister, daughter, career woman. But when you scratched the surface, things fell apart quickly.

Perhaps Sam was offering a way to cut through the intellect and get right to the core. Using touch to bring body and mind and emotions together made intuitive sense. What could be bad about finding yourself while experiencing pleasure? I hadn't known that was even an option.

Sam wasn't one of the swashbucklers I fancied, but maybe he held the promise of something more than ripped muscles. (Besides, I could always close my eyes.) I called and confirmed. I was in.

Chapter Eight

Queens and Tigers and Pam, Oh My

The following Tuesday I made sure my cousin Sophia would be stationed across the street from Sam's Upper West Side apartment. She was the only one of the gang I'd invited to watch my back that night. She thought I was hilarious, sure, but not crazy, and she was my cheerleader in a way that the others weren't. She understood what it was to live an off-the-beaten-track life—she dated African-American men when it was a rarity; managed to remain close friends with her ex-husband; her dentist was an ex-lover; and she now lived happily with her girlfriend, Joan. Sophia was fearless and accepting, without a judgmental bone in her body. She was the one who urged me to stick with in vitro fertilization when everyone else thought it was a science experiment. "It's your only chance of having your baby?" I remembered her asking. "Then you've gotta take it." In its own way, this was no different. Sophia got it.

On Sam day, I shaved and creamed and mani-pedied, exactly as if I were prepping for the gynecologist. I dressed without hesitation, pulling on an Eileen Fisher coordinated denim ensemble with slimming jeans and a short jacket, black Lucchese boots, and a string of turquoise stones around my neck. Urban cowboy meets suburban housewife.

I left enough time to find free street parking because I needed to start saving my pennies. If sensual massage worked for me as well as it did for Ricky, I could see it becoming an expensive habit. The buzzer unlocked the front door the second I pushed the bell. I guessed Sam was antsy, this being a first for him, too.

I climbed five steamy flights, looking for the familiar face. The only person I saw was an older guy in baggy running shorts, a faded tee, and bright green sweat socks leaning over the banister, his eyes fixed on the stairwell. I paused on the landing below, squinting up at the diminutive man who had at least fifteen years on the dude in the photo.

"Sam?"

I wasn't expecting Hugh Jackman, but I wasn't expecting Señor Senior, either.

"Pam! A pleasure. Welcome. Come on in."

I so didn't want to, but I retreated into politeness and followed his footsteps. I wondered whether he intentionally pulled a bait and switch or whether he just didn't get that Mother Nature is relentless.

I craved a big, powerful guy who could easily wrap his hands around my "full-figured" body. I doubted Sam's hands could span my wrist. At least I didn't have to worry about safety. I could take him if I had to.

We sat in his homey, spacious living room decorated with personal artifacts. He poured ice water from a vintage pitcher into a matching glass and asked if I wanted a slice of lemon. This was so much harder than being at SoHo Touch, way more intimate.

"What brings you to this session?" Sam asked, the consummate professional.

"Well, I'm not sure I'm staying yet." The words came out in an unconscious rush. My own insensitivity was embarrassing. I tried to cover the lapse with a smile.

He steamed ahead. "I can tell you're feeling really nervous. If it helps, Pam, I can tell you I am, too. I promise it's worth it. There's so much you can learn through your body."

Sam's efforts to put me at ease were heroic, but his inexperience with women loomed as large as the massage table in the next room. He was saying all the right things, but my body wasn't listening. I wanted to bolt, but I was trapped into staying by his goodwill and my good manners. I was going to get my safe and contained, non-threatening "erotic" experience whether I wanted it or not.

"Do you want me to be naked during the massage?" Sam inquired matter-of-factly.

"NO! No. Really. Thank you. No."

Undeterred, he let me know that if I wanted to touch him, that that was okay, too.

Touch him? Why would I want to do that? It never occurred to me. He's supposed to touch me. Who said anything about interactivity?

"No thanks, I'm good."

"I'm very good at anal massage," he said. "Would you be open to that experience?"

"Um, well, I'm open to touch, so I guess, um, we could see how it goes?"

I made a short trip to the bathroom before we got down to it. There was a big gilt *Q* on the door. Q? Q! Q for Queen! Perfect, two queens and not a king for miles.

I'd barely gotten settled on the table when the oil rained down on my back. What is it with sensual massage guys and grease? At least Sam had fantastic, experienced hands that made me relax the minute he started.

Sam went over my back and buttocks and legs, and before I knew it, he had maneuvered me into that spread frog position. Let me tell you, nothing opens you up faster than thighs pushed apart. Talk about vulnerable.

Sam's fingers were exploring my nether regions where no man, except Gavin, had gone before. Damn. I almost allowed myself to stop thinking and relax into pure feeling. It felt good—not erotic, but sensual. My anus purred. *Forty-three years. Why'd you wait so long?* I asked myself. Right away, the obvious litany of answers popped up: fear, ignorance, convention, and shame.

But, as Sam softly touched the flesh of my bottom, the much harder question pushed its way into my brain. Why had I been so resistant to pleasure just for me all these years? Sure, I had a monthly massage. But I couldn't even justify window-shopping for myself without buying things for the kids or Gavin. I didn't think I deserved it. Sam's hands seemed to be making the point that this pleasure, when I could let myself feel it, was exclusively for me.

I was drifting into deeper reverie when Sam's voice interrupted.

"Would you turn over, please," he requested. I did and was almost knocked off the table by the shock waves of his anxiety as he faced my female parts. After all, everyone has an asshole. That was a well-mapped area for him. This was uncharted territory. I could see him trying to make friends with my vulva, gingerly laying his hands over the outside. I imagined him poring over *Gray's Anatomy* before the session. I was beginning to doubt whether it was possible for a hetero woman and a gay man to generate sensual heat together.

And I was doomed to give another gay man at least one shot. I had answered an e-mail that came in that morning from "Tantric Tiger." One look at his picture and I had booked for the next day. So maybe I was superficial. What can I say? The Tiger's looks turned me on. Sam's did not. It wasn't like there was much beyond looks to go on. Their Web sites used similar holistic, crunchy granola language. They made erotic touch sound wholesome. It made sense to me that I'd hang my final decision on the image of a face and body that fed my fantasies.

I tried to tune out the noise in my head and focus on this moment and Sam's hands. My body felt awake, a little confused, and definitely not turned on. The clock had run out, which was fine because I was done.

"You were such a brave girl with your first anal massage," Sam praised me gently.

It was only proper to return the compliment. "Thank you. You were a great, uh, anal massager."

I got dressed and paid my bill. As I was finding my way to the door his bouncing, hairy, designer-hybrid dog escaped the bedroom. "Down! Get down!" Sam's shouts provoked the dog to madness. "I said get down, Samson! SAMSON!"

Samson? C'mon. Really?

I almost split my seams holding it together until I ran out onto the street and into Sophia's waiting arms. I didn't have a second to catch my breath before Sophia began to pepper me with a thousand questions on the way to a neighborhood tavern. The Upper West Side is littered with every kind of trendy restaurant, but this place can't be beat for a down-home dirty martini and burger—my idea of mother's milk. The second we slid into the cracked leatherette banquette, I started spilling.

"Sophia, what are you doing tomorrow night?" I began.

"I have to check my calendar. I think I promised Joan we'd go to a Yankees game. Why?"

"I have something to tell you."

"Did that shit hurt you? I'll kill him," my protector said, waving a balled fist. "What's going on?"

"No, no. My God, Sam is the sweetest queen you'll ever meet," I said after we ordered from an improbably handsome young waiter. I waited for the martinis to show up and the first sip of Grey Goose to hit my veins. "I booked another appointment."

Sophia's face went through a dozen expressions in less than thirty seconds. "You're kidding, right? Another session? With this guy?" She belted back half her drink. "Are you out of your mind?"

"Well, maybe. But no, not with Sam. I booked a different masseur. He answered my e-mail, too. He was really warm and together . . . unlike the guy who told me he'd be glad to spin me around on his cock. Which I think is way too advanced for me."

An 80-proof stream spewed from Sophia's side of the table. "Wow, elementary cock spinning. Honey, what are you getting into?"

"I didn't answer him. I'm talking about the Tantric Tiger. I checked his Web site. He's a total pro and his picture is to die for. He's all about moving deep inside yourself and finding your own inner pleasure. He called it 'waking up your sleeping beauty.' He could be the prince I want to wake me up."

I thought about Tantric Tiger. Markus was his real name. Tripping through his site that morning was like wandering a carefully tended garden blooming with tenderness, spirituality, and sensuality. His tone and approach, his boyish, beautiful face and lean body: It was the total package. I dialed the number and spoke directly to the Tiger. Yes, he had worked on one or two women in the past. He mostly worked on men, but he was happy to work with me.

I went through my spiel about monogamy and fidelity and chewed my cuticle while I waited for him to think it over. I was in an eerily familiar state of suspension. In those seconds, I flashed back to the anxious wait after each pregnancy test. There had been so many letdowns before Gavin and I finally conceived. I got good at steeling myself against disappointment. While I hung on the line, I realized I'd already prepared myself for the Tiger's "no."

"I get it," he said at last. "You don't want to wake up one morning when you're eighty and think, 'Oh, I could have had a V8!' Of course, I'd be delighted to work with you."

And just like that, I was hooked. Even though I thought it might be a bit much to have two massages in two days, the Tiger was a bonbon. And I do love my sweets.

Sophia hooted. "I'll be there when you get out even if it means missing Derek Jeter. Joan is gonna kill me. But I gotta see your face when I debrief you. Honey, you're a riot. How fa-a-abulous. I'm gonna ask Vicki to hang with me. I need a witness."

Without hesitation, I agreed. Truth? Being the center of attention this way was a rush. It felt big and spicy. For once, I was the sex kitten, not Vicki, my Woodstocky, once-upon-a-time free-love sister.

"Tomorrow at four p.m. Tantric Tiger's studio is in midtown on the East Side. I'll e-mail the address. Boy oh boy. I just might get myself a V8. Gr-r-r-r."

Chapter Nine

The Year of the Tiger

I DOUBLE-CHECKED THE HOUSE before I left for the Tiger's lair. I'd baked a fresh lasagna for Gavin and the boys and left precise heating instructions stuck to the fridge. I had to do right by my men. Not that I felt the least bit conscience-stricken. I had had a couple of overpriced, vaguely risqué massages. Big deal. So far, my big, fat sex adventures hadn't rocked my world. There were moments, though, that piqued my curiosity.

I'd indulged in my ritual cleansing and dressing, made sure the gas was off and a living-room light turned on. By the time I hit the road to midtown Manhattan, it was rush hour and the toll lane was jammed.

"Shit," I shouted. "I'm gonna be late."

Fishing around in my bag for change for the toll, I pulled out a dollar bill. Stuck to it was a photo my mother had given me the day before.

It was an ancient Kodak. Me at one of Great Neck's ultraexclusive private pools. I was maybe four or five years old, a sylph in a tiger-striped bikini and giant lifeguard boots.

"Look at you posing like that. You were a precocious little thing, Pammy. So cute," Mom had reminisced, thrusting the photo at me.

Yeah, well, that was then. I jammed the fading picture back into my purse, the image burned into my brain. I *was* cute. Where'd that girl go? That photo was evidence that there was a time when I was comfortable and confident in my body. Not self-conscious in the least. Just being.

That was gone by the time I was ten and my mother was dragging me to the plus-size stores. That maiden voyage to Lane Bryant sent the first public message that I didn't fit in, that I wasn't the right size. All my friends were in hip-huggers and tiny psychedelic tank tops, while I dressed in the matronly stretch polyester coordinates, the "husky girl" wardrobe staple.

Now, as I waited in the conga line of cars, I kept thinking about my five-year-old open smile and I teared up. I don't remember ever again feeling that uninhibited in my own skin.

Well, I told myself, *move on. Yesterday is so over.* I concentrated on Markus and the new Tiger stripes I was going to have. But the closer I got to midtown, the more intrusive the repressed Pam grew. The old tape began to loop. I knew it so well I could sing along. *You're too large, we don't have that in your size, the plus section is over there. Those pants aren't really cut for you, dear.* I instinctively checked the backseat to see if my kids had left an open bag of chips or a half-eaten cookie, anything to soothe the anxiety. I found nothing to distract me from the voices in my head. The volume was only getting louder.

Who did this stuff, anyway? Who e-mailed unknown men and arranged for sensual massages? What straight woman visited a gay Web site looking for a service that didn't seem to exist? Part of me knew it was lunacy. And part of me, a deep part, felt like I was on a mission to save myself from the hunger that was eating me alive. God knows I'd tried to satisfy the beast. I was classic, eating my way through bags of pretzels and hunks of cheese, and beating myself up for the unacceptable behavior and overweight, overwrought results. Clearly, I was famished, ravenous for something that food couldn't satisfy. I reached into my bag again for the old bikini photo and knew that it was somehow connected to a primal yearning that was at the bursting point.

By the time I found a parking spot and walked into Markus's handsome building, I was late. A brawny, elegantly outfitted doorman announced me. Fighting down waves of fear, I took the elevator to the fourteenth floor.

"This way," a warm voice rang out as the elevator doors hissed open. I followed it around the hallway corner and there he was. Markus looked exactly like his photo, only better. He was blond and tan, wearing a sarong low on his narrow hips and a dozen beaded necklaces on his bare chest.

Markus was a beautiful jungle boy, which only torqued my anxiety. He was so much closer to everything I thought I wanted. Markus had heartthrob energy.

He walked me into his vine-draped, orchid-filled living room. The wide-open door framed a rare Manhattan terrace, covered in flourishing bamboo and morning glories. He settled me into a chair that directly faced his own.

No small talk. The Tiger wanted to know things, real things. What was I seeking? Was I loved at home? Did I receive touch? Did I love my husband? Did my husband know that I was here with him?

I was getting sick of that last question. Every person I had told about my nascent adventure had asked me if Gavin knew what I was doing.

"No," I said. "He doesn't. I don't have the words to tell myself, let alone Gavin, what I'm doing here."

I explained one more time that this was about me, not my husband or my marriage. I loved that Gavin loved me the way I was, for decades. That's a lot of different hairstyles. But I had no concept of my sexuality, my femaleness outside of marriage to this one man. I existed erotically only as a reflection in his eyes. I had no way of knowing myself outside of that.

"I never brought my husband into my psychotherapy sessions and I feel the same way about this. I plan to tell him one day, but I need to know what I'm doing first. And I don't, not yet."

Tiger kept firing questions. I managed to answer them without withholding a thing.

"I'm afraid that if I don't explore that side of me, I'll explode. I'm terrified that if I do explore it, I'll explode. I don't know what to do. And I think I disguise my fear as boredom. My husband is a fine lover. It's not him. It's me. Something deep I don't know how to name."

Markus nodded this time, giving me room to go on.

"I feel sexually alive, but I don't know how to bring that out. It's not that I want to bring it out. It's more that I need to. I'm tired of trying to eat my way out of boredom. And frustration."

"It sounds to me like you're a caged bird, pulling out your own feathers to keep your mind occupied," Markus said.

That struck deep. It was true. I hurt myself instead of letting myself be. Overeating was my weapon of choice. My weight was my battle scar. While we were talking about my food demons, I could not stop staring at the Tiger. Markus was slender, tight, and toned. I wasn't, and it was making me even more self-conscious. *Oh God, I am fat,* the old tape droned. *Why didn't I crash-diet before I started this? He is going to see my stomach. Why did I fall off Jenny Craig, Weight Watchers, South Beach, and Atkins?*

Markus picked up on my agitation and asked if he could rub my feet while we talked. I slipped off my sandal and offered him a perfectly pedicured foot. He cradled it in his warm, strong hands.

After about half an hour, the Tiger asked me to stand up and look directly into his eyes. "Eye gazing," he called it. I did it, but the intimacy made me squirm. I had to fight the urge to look away. What was I afraid he would see in me?

"Could we please just get started?" I asked, breaking the gaze.

"We already did. We are in the session," Markus answered. "But if you'd like to start the massage, we certainly can."

"Yes, please. I really would."

He removed the screen that hid his work area. I freaked out. There wasn't the usual and expected massage table. Only a futon on the floor covered in flower petals. Were those pink rose petals for me? An entire butterfly farm took flight in my belly. I had no idea what this was all about.

Markus told me to get undressed and stepped into another room. Now, undressing was something I could do. I'd been doing it so often lately, I could almost ignore the usual litany of critical observations as I pulled off my clothes. I was down to the buff before noticing there wasn't a towel. I needed cover.

"Markus, do you have a towel or a sheet?" I asked, holding my shirt up to cover my nakedness.

"Why?" the Tiger demanded softly. "If you want one, that's okay. But honey, I'm going to be seeing all of you in a minute." He came back in, flashed a mischievous grin, and handed me a towel.

Was I really going to be naked with this man? Was he going to touch my body? I couldn't think straight. I got on the futon, stomach down, and covered my bottom. I tried to act like this was any other massage. I closed my eyes, told myself I was safe, and pretended that I wasn't in this body.

I told myself I could leave at any time. Sophia and Vicki were right downstairs keeping a lookout.

Before I could get any more lost in my head, I sensed Markus right beside me. I could smell him. Herbs and spices. Exotic scents like I imagined I'd find in a market in India. It almost made me drunk. He put a steadying hand on my back and the air filled my lungs again. Until he rolled me over. Good Christ! Was he naked?

My eyes quickly scanned all of him. He was more than naked. He was beautifully naked. Gorgeously naked. Spectacularly naked. I thought I'd jump out of my skin. Oh! My! God! His skin was so golden! He had no tan lines. Even his cock was tan. I hadn't seen a stomach that flat in a million years. Why was he naked? What was he going to do to me? What the hell was he planning? We'd never discussed the possibility of his nudity. I didn't ask for it.

I lifted my head and looked into his eyes. I calmed down.

He's gay, Pam. He is so gay and you are so not a man.

Markus laid a small, soft, lavender-filled pillow over my eyes, blocking out the Adonis. Anxious and wide-awake, I began to feel his hands run over my body. This time there was no oil, only a soft powder drifting over my skin, like snowdrops. He told me that I smelled good, like a tropical flower. It made me happy in some girlie way.

His hands made contact with my flesh again. Then something sandpapery teased my breasts. What was that? Was that his chin stubble? Whoa! I wasn't expecting that, either. Soon I was gasping and sweating as Markus touched me, murmuring into my ear.

"You have such a healthy, beautiful body," he told me. He chanted it so many times I started to believe it, allowing in bits of reassurance, letting go just a little of the old body hatred.

I must have been very quiet because Markus said, "You get five extra minutes for every sound you make. You get free time for every noise. Let me know that you're enjoying the touch."

I let some sound escape and, like a twisted soccer mom, Markus cheered me with an "attagirl." I finally let myself enjoy the unfamiliar feelings that ran through me. He kept reminding me to breathe, demonstrating the technique, helping me to keep the air flowing, the sounds coming.

The thrill in my body was so intense that I thought I might go into cardiac arrest. People did die from too much sexual excitement, right?

He may have spent most of his professional time on men, but Markus knew exactly how and where to touch me. Between breaths, I noticed that my mind had stopped nattering and I was in a trance of rapture. It crowded out everything else. I had no idea something like this was possible without actually making love.

I climaxed.

Oh shit. I had an orgasm with someone other than my husband. It was unbearably exciting and unimaginably intense. I was shocked. After Sam and Boris, I didn't know what to expect. Who was this man? How could I have such a private moment with a stranger?

Markus uncovered my eyes and offered me a dainty cup filled with jasmine green tea.

"Welcome back, sweetheart. Why don't you rest for a few minutes? Don't rush. Get dressed whenever you feel ready," he said and left me to "Sail Away" with Enya.

I sailed right into denial. I put on my clothes as fast as I could.

"Thank you so much for that massage. It was better than anything I had at Bliss," I mumbled, flying out the door as fast as my wedges would allow.

Vicki and Sophia rushed the doorman and grabbed me in a huddle right in the lobby. I wanted to blurt it all out, but didn't dare say a word until we were outside. I already suspected the doorman took one look at my uncombed hair and knew exactly what I'd been up to.

Sophia held me at arm's length and carefully studied my face. "Oh my," she said. "Look at you. You look great."

"And your shirt's on inside out," Vicki said dryly.

Chapter Ten

Home Again

GETTING BACK TO Riverdale was endless. Markus had taken the starch out of me. Sophia and Vicki interrogated me remorselessly about every moment of those three Tiger hours. They wanted it in glorious Technicolor and CinemaScope, over a drinkable dinner.

"How come you're not eating? You must be starving after all that activity," Vicki worried.

I was well into my second glass of cabernet when I realized I had no desire for food. Interesting. "No, really. I'm fine. Great, as a matter of fact."

We got back to the real subject of our dinner.

"Not even a G-string?"

"He rubbed his stubble *where*?"

They asked me to repeat the good stuff so many times I started to feel like it had happened to someone else.

"When I saw the futon and no massage table, I was scared. After the first two minutes, though, I felt safe. The Tiger operates in a different world than Boris or Sam. Even his sandalwood and cinnamon smell excited me. But he definitely took me on a roller-coaster ride.

He made me feel like I was a princess and then pushed me to my edges." Markus knew how to coach me into having pleasure in a way that was different than anything I'd experienced before. It wasn't about the lover. It was about me. I didn't have to think about whether he was enjoying himself or if it was his turn. It was extraordinary.

"He was genuinely earnest about the healing stuff, and omigod does he ever know how to touch a woman. It was ecstatic."

"C'mon. Ecstatic? That must've been some orgasm," Vicki said.

"It wasn't about the orgasm. That was a bonus. It was the freedom to just experience pleasure."

Two hours of vicarious erotic massage later, they let me go. After I paid the parking-lot ransom and got behind the wheel, the realities of Riverdale sobered me faster than a cold shower and a gallon of coffee. I wasn't ready for real life. I'd finally had a full-blown sex-goddess moment and I was in no mood to strike the wife-and-mother pose, chat about a lost science project or my in-laws' latest high-seas high jinks.

I was glad I had made it a late night with my girls. I was certain—or at least certainly hoping—that Gavin and the boys were asleep. A small pang of guilt got me, but only because I didn't feel guiltier that I'd had my V8 and liked it so much I wanted to lick the glass clean. I knew that this was outside the box and there'd be people who, if they knew, would insist I should feel bad. There would be judgment and I'd be labeled "unfaithful." No matter what anyone else thought, I didn't call what happened cheating.

I was still traveling light-years away from my everyday life as I pulled up in front of my building. At this moment, my body was the center of my universe. When was the last time I felt my body? I mean, really felt all of my parts? When was the last time I felt this alive? When was the last time I felt such deep pleasure?

Not since I was a newlywed, when just Gavin's touch on my

nipples brought the house down. He was and is a tender lover. He cared more about my orgasm than he did about his own. Gavin was like that about everything. He taught my boys to hold doors open and help our neighbors with their grocery bags. Gavin also made me feel tended to in our daily life. But that had nothing to do with what I was experiencing now.

I parked in our building's garage and took the elevator to the fifth floor. I turned my key in the apartment lock, anticipating the familiar chaos. Everything was exactly the way it was every night.

I didn't bother to clean up. I didn't care.

I tiptoed into the bedroom. Gavin was fast asleep. I undressed quietly and slid under the covers. I felt Gavin's warmth. He must have felt mine because his hand reached for me instinctively. I folded myself around him the way I had every night for the past twenty-five years. We always nestled like two spoons. And out of nowhere, fear took me. I loved this man deeply and I wanted nothing to come between us. Up until this evening, nothing ever had. But now I'd had a life-altering experience and I wasn't sharing it with him. Sam and Boris, the computer search—all that felt like kiddie pranks. This? This was big, and I couldn't let it go.

I was sure another tectonic plate had shifted.

I couldn't keep this a secret from Gavin, but I couldn't imagine telling him. How could I explain that my body had been asleep in a glass box without hurting him? He took pride in being my good lover. How could he ever understand that a gay prince in a flowered sarong had awakened me, not with a kiss but by asking me to close my eyes and do nothing but feel? How could he get it when even I couldn't grasp it yet?

There was one thing I knew for sure: I was going back for more.

I burrowed deeper into my beloved's body and willed myself to sleep.

Chapter Eleven

An Unexpected Geisha

Two days later I was giddy with desire for another session, but I could see that if I wasn't careful my pleasure hunt would gut my family's finances. What was I going to do, swap out fresh steaks and greens for canned chili and hope they didn't notice? "No, my darlings. No second helpings of beans and rice for you. You know Mummy loves you, but she must see the Tantric Tiger or she will eat her young."

Then there was the whole protocol thing. I already wanted to see Markus again, but wasn't that just slutty? He had asked me to call to let him know how I was doing, so I figured I'd just slip the question into our conversation. He was the expert. I waited another day, then dialed.

"It's me, Pam. Pamela Madsen. I wanted to let you know I'm feeling good, more connected to my body. I'm breathing more consciously and, by the way, do you have time to see me next week?"

So much for subtle.

"Already?" I could hear the smile.

I was a slut.

"Is it too soon? If it is, really, I can wait. No problem. Honestly . . ."

"No," he said, laughing. "It's not too soon. It's just that men don't often come back so quickly."

Well, I thought, *men can be so stupid.*

Next Wednesday rolled around and I was in a new state of mind. I ditched the backup squad. I told Beth I was seeing Markus again, and she offered to stand guard, but I made her settle for a postsession check-in. I was launched and I needed to see how I flew solo.

"Do you self-pleasure?" Markus inquired matter-of-factly the minute I was seated. I almost fell out of my chair.

"Excuse me?" The blood was rising to my cheeks, and I don't blush easily.

"Do you self-pleasure?" he repeated in a calm, steady voice.

"Um, er, well, no. Yes. I do. Sometimes. Not very often," I stuttered. "Unless 'self-pleasure' means masturbation. In that case, yes, I do."

"Do you use your hands? A vibrator? How do you self-pleasure?"

Jeez. Self-pleasure? My hands? A vibrator? Did he really need to know this to give me a massage?

"Both," I muttered, and took a swig of water from the bottle labeled I'M BEAUTIFUL that he'd thoughtfully provided.

"Do you have orgasms when you self-pleasure?" he inquired.

"Yes, I do. Sometimes more than one."

Without skipping a beat, he asked, "What do you fantasize about when you self-pleasure?"

My back stiffened. I never talked about my fantasies, not even with my husband. I could hardly admit them to myself. There was no way I could say them out loud to this man. I punted.

"I remember a time when I was about ten and I first started to masturbate. I had orgasms. I didn't know what they were. They just felt so good. I remember getting lost in the sensation. And I remember playing music. That's what it was. The music. It carried me through the waves of a kind of mindless pleasure. I don't feel that now. Fantasy. Vibrators. They don't do it. I guess I was freer then."

"Goddess, how do you feel about your body?"

Oh no. More talking. I was paying for touch. My body? I didn't love that topic. What was there to say? I needed to lose at least sixty pounds. I was a size 16, depending on the day and the designer.

Markus probed further, adjusting his sarong, crossing his legs, settling in. "What are the parts of your body that you like?"

I swallowed the mortification and managed to say something kind about my full breasts. "I like that despite nursing two children, my breasts don't sag or hang," I whispered. At least, I don't think they do. It's been a long time since I actually looked at them. Then I ventured, "I like my round, firm bottom and my face and hair." I looked at his open face and was seized by candor. "I don't have an easy relationship with my body. I've always struggled with my weight. I don't like my body. Some days, I really, really hate it." Tears began trickling down my cheeks.

"Maybe I was eleven, maybe I was nine—somewhere in there, I'm not sure. I found raspberries in a bowl in the refrigerator. They were the kind frozen in syrup that you had to defrost before you could eat them. I took some. I remember the rush of cold and sweet. I told my mother how much I loved them. She wheeled on me with such anger I thought I'd die.

"'They are not for chubby girls like you!' she screamed in my face, ranting. 'They're for your brother. You know he's getting over ulcer surgery! How could you eat them?'"

A cry convulsed me. "I loved those raspberries," I sobbed to Markus. "I was so hurt. My mother always had the same devastating message: I was too fat for anything good. The good stuff wasn't for me."

The Tiger discreetly kept the tissues coming while I blubbered. "That was my first true memory of food being forbidden to me because of my size."

I ran out of words. Markus waited while the hurricane of memory and emotion blew over.

"Starting today, Pam, I want you to look at your naked body every day and touch yourself and tell yourself beautiful things about all your parts," the Tiger instructed.

As fucking if! I couldn't think of anything more horrible. I wasn't going to do this. Absolutely not! As far as I was concerned, I didn't exist in the mirror below the neck. I carefully avoided all full-length mirrors unless I was fully clothed in the camouflage outfits I'd perfected. Thank God fashion for fat girls had come a long way. Designers discovered an untapped niche in us big gals who feign self-acceptance. I had a wardrobe full of dramatic capes and long, loose sweaters in luxe fabrics. I had an extraordinary collection of fabulous earrings that guided the viewer's attention right to my "pretty face" and dramatic dark hair. After all this effort, he wanted me to look at what I'd so masterfully disguised. I didn't think I could face that reality.

"Now I'm going to touch you," Markus said.

Was this his idea of foreplay? I was ready to run.

"Pamela, relax. We're going to pretend that you're fifteen and have never been touched before," he said as he pulled me to my feet. He drew me so close to his body that I could feel his warm breath on my neck.

"Princess, I am going to ask you to close your eyes and keep them shut. Can you do that for me?" I shook with nerves and excitement. I nodded.

The Tiger started to touch my body while we were standing together. He awakened me with gentle pressure on my arm, my belly, and my back. "May I remove your clothing?" I moaned as the blouse, pants, and shame fell away. All the while, he stroked and caressed me everywhere. Markus moved me into the trance state I had found the first time with him. His touch brought me out of my always-wrong body to my having no body at all. I was pure sensation, erotic thoughtlessness. He took me firmly by the arm and guided me around the apartment, asking me to step up and then down. I realized he was easing me into a tub of warm, fragrant water.

When did he get this ready for me? How did he know I loved baths? He drizzled the water over my shoulders, my back, and my breasts. Nobody had ever done that for me that I could remember. Markus was washing all of me, touching me in places I didn't know were so charged they could take me to the brink. He used sponges, his hands, a loofah. I had no choice but to surrender to the bliss. The very act of bathing made my unworthy body feel worthy, deserving, and precious. He took my hand, tenderly lifting me, newly baptized, out of the tub, and he softly dried me before he placed me on the familiar futon.

Markus cranked the music, abruptly shifting the mood in the room. The beat throbbed. My geisha was turning back into a playful tiger. He blew air bubbles on my belly, making me giggle and filling me with joy. I felt spicy and beautiful. Imagine. He made me feel like a sex kitten. I felt so free. His hands massaged me, played with me, teased me. The music carried me deep into myself and I welcomed it. My secret fantasies didn't even enter my mind. Just like when I was a child, I rode the waves of music into long, rolling orgasms that went on and on. The gift of it stunned me. I had wanted that back for so long. I had tried over the years, but I could never reach that innocent ecstasy. As a grown-up, I had to retreat into fantasy, romance novels, and porn. What Markus gave me was like a meditation. I was flying through the universe filled with bright color.

Tantric Tiger was a genius.

Chapter Twelve

She Wore a Raspberry Beret

I FORCED MYSELF TO do Markus's look-touch-say exercise every day as soon as the apartment emptied out. I hated it, but I owed Markus at least a good faith effort. I had one full-length mirror in my house, nailed to the inside of my closet door, that I used only for a quick once-over to make sure my skirt wasn't tucked into my pantyhose before I left the house. I never spent more than thirty seconds in front of it. I had my cultivated look down cold. I didn't need a mirror. Standing naked and staring into one was torture, even for a second. Two minutes would leave me dead. I broke the exercise down into parts.

I went topless first. I was relieved that my memory of my still-buoyant breasts was pretty accurate. So I said nice things to them out loud. I gave them a "positive affirmation" the way the homework sheet told me to. "Lookin' good, girls."

I tried to "breathe into" the fact that my solid arms were starting to show signs of cottage cheese and sag. I couldn't. My mother's perimenopause speech filled my head. *You know, Pamela, it's not too late. You could firm those up. My Jane Fonda tapes and twenty pounds would make all the difference.*

I closed the closet door.

The effort left me so raw, the dam burst immediately the next time I sat in Markus's stupid check-in chairs. Out came the same litany of wrong.

"I can never be the right size. I never have the right look. I'm so sick of it."

This wasn't psychoanalysis, but you sure could have fooled me. My nose ran, mascara bled down my face, my hair clung to my cheeks. Lovely. I couldn't stop the boo-hooing. Markus, with practiced dispassion, asked me to go on.

"No matter how successful I am, it always feels like my true success is measured by how fat or thin I am that day. It doesn't matter that I helped pass laws so that insurance companies can't deny fertility patients treatment. None of it matters. I'm always inadequate because I'm too much."

Once again, the Tiger waited for me to wind down. "This is good. It's expected. The whole point of Sacred Intimacy is that it's a sexual path to self," he explained. "It consciously uses erotic energy to trigger its transformative and therapeutic potential."

Here I thought I was coming for two hours of jungle boy and instead got Sigmund Freud in a sarong. "You should read Joseph Kramer, the SI founder. You'd find it so illuminating."

To put theory into practice, Markus asked me if I could surrender all that negative feeling and just be in my body. Surrender? I loved that word when he said it. So sexy. It jump-started me.

Markus got up from his chair and walked over to me, heavy coral beads clacking against his tawny chest. He bent down, put his arms around me, and said, "Can you give up your self-judgment for ninety minutes?" I nodded. "Goddess, this is what Sacred Intimacy is all about. I'd like to blindfold you," he whispered.

"Say wha'?" I croaked. So long, Freud; hello, Tiger.

I mulled it over, wiping my makeup-streaked face. Blindfold, huh? That scared me a little. It kind of excited me, too. A blindfold was different than the eye pillow he'd used before. It smacked of something taboo and it thrilled me. I don't know why it didn't occur to me that I could just take it off, but it didn't. I went with it.

While I lay naked on the futon, Markus arranged me on the center of the mat and tied a piece of black silk around my eyes. I could hear my heart pound. "Just feel, princess. Don't think. Just feel the beauty of your body," he whispered.

I felt a brush of air over my skin as a new scent wrapped my body. Markus was burning incense, fanning it over me. I felt like an offering to the gods. In a Tiger ritual, he applied tiny drops of delicately scented oil to my feet, my back, my bottom. Goose bumps of anticipation covered my flesh.

Markus placed my arms by my sides. "Keep them there unless I ask you to move." The Tiger's voice was deep and throaty.

He was asking me to listen, to receive and follow directions. For a woman who was used to leading, passivity was strange and difficult.

And then the touch began. Slowly, Markus massaged my body so deeply that it hurt in places. When I protested he commanded me, "Be still. Breathe."

He kneaded and stretched me, and when I was a puddle of soft flesh, I felt him gently blowing on my skin.

Oh God. Then soft tickles, then light drumbeats over my buttocks and down my legs. A groan escaped as the breath, the tickles, and the teasing spanks played over every part of me.

Oh yes. This was certainly spiritual! I was praying to God with every ounce of my being. I was aflame as Markus's hands moved into my yielding, warm recesses. It was hard not to move. The blindfold made me feel vulnerable. But in truth, the excitement of pure submission and surrender blotted out everything else.

His dominance allowed me to just let go and feel. There was so much sensation, I couldn't be anywhere else but right here in this moment, I couldn't think about anything other than what was happening to me right now. It was a revelation. This ecstasy was foreign and profound, and it lasted so long that I thought I was going to die. My friends would have to come and get my body, dress it, and dump it in a remote landfill somewhere in Jersey.

When Markus decided that this quivering mass of cytoplasm had had enough, he gently wrapped me in a sheet and told me to rest. "I'll be right back."

I floated. I don't know for how long. Maybe five minutes, maybe two days. He removed my blindfold and I blinked in the dim candlelight. He gathered me so that my body and his were very close on the mat. I was still foggy when he asked me to open my mouth.

"Huh?"

"Just open your mouth," he softly ordered. So I did. And a taste as old as childhood filled my mouth. Sweet. Frozen. Forbidden. Raspberries. The juice ran from the corners of my mouth and my eyes welled with tears.

"The raspberries are always there for you," Markus said. "They're meant for you, anytime you want. Just reach for them."

Chapter Thirteen

Homework

Things were starting to shift in my world. This Riverdale housewife had a new spring to her step. Doormen saluted me with an enthusiastic "Good morning!" and followed me with their eyes when I passed. That hadn't happened in years. I smiled right back at them, giving my hair a flirty toss and making eye contact. I was feeling bold and sexy all the time. It was dawning on me that feeling sexy made me sexy. And I hadn't lost a single pound.

Everyone noticed there was something new about Pamela. Everyone except Gavin. As far as I could tell, he was oblivious, and that was just fine with me. I enjoyed having a dark secret. Sure, there were moments when I wanted to tell him everything. I had never kept anything from him before, and sometimes I struggled with it in the middle of the night. Fear kept my lips sealed. I was afraid that he wouldn't understand, or that he'd judge me, or most of all, that he'd shut me down. That, I couldn't bear. His anger, eh, I could handle that. But the possibility of losing what I had just begun to find in myself was unimaginable.

I was learning how to reclaim my sense of myself as a woman. Markus wasn't merely a master of sensual massage; he ran an erotic rehab center. He was teaching me how to tune out all the voices and learn to experience myself in each moment. At first, I resented the mirror homework. But I kept at it because I knew Markus was helping me pry open another padlocked door.

Every day I doggedly peeled away another garment and faced my round, earth mother reflection. I graduated to touching myself as I watched my body respond. I let my hands stray all over and I told each part loving and caring things. I lied.

Within a few weeks, I was softening toward myself until I could take in the whole, entirely buff me. The reflected image resembled a woman of the Renaissance. I thought about all the museums I'd ever visited where my body type was on display in hundreds of years' worth of paintings and sculptures—the epitome of the feminine ideal.

I thanked Markus every day for opening my eyes. During one session, the Tiger swaddled me in a sheet and began to massage me through the covers. His hands were powerful. His exotic smells permeated every fiber in his studio and infiltrated my senses. Music, deep and tribal, started to play.

"You are entitled to all the love and pleasure in the universe, princess. You are beautiful and deserving just the way you are." Markus's voice was throaty, his mouth right against my ear. "Breathe!"

He kneaded and lengthened my muscles, awakened me with soft touches that drifted by my nipples and inner thighs. I was melting. "Give me sounds," Markus said. "A dollar for every noise! Let me hear your pleasure!" Soon I was moaning with abandon.

With my eyes shut tightly, he led me into the sensual trance I craved. Who knew that a foot could be tickled in so many ways? I was a shameless sponge. My body exploded in climax. I was ready to cover up and drift.

Markus was not having it. He kept me tethered to him, opened up and receiving. "Come on. I know you can give me more than that."

I did, over and over again, until Markus wrapped me in a silk sheet and rocked me to a soft landing. He rolled me on my side and lay behind me.

"Open your eyes, kitten. Open them."

Reluctant to relinquish the darkness, I did. What I saw horrified me. Markus had positioned a full-length mirror so that it reflected every ounce of me. I closed my eyes tight.

"Come on, sweetheart. It isn't so bad. Let's look together. Just for a minute!"

No. I didn't want to do that. He couldn't make me. Wasn't it time to go home? But it was clear that I wasn't getting my panties back until I obeyed.

It had been hard enough to do this by myself. Having a witness was torment. Unwillingly, I opened one eye a slit and was shocked at my own beauty. I was exactly like the reclining goddess in Rousseau's iconic painting *The Dream,* resting on my side with my long black hair draping my face.

After that day, I began to use different measures of beauty. When I looked in the mirror, I was lying less and less to my arms, my stomach, my hips, and my thighs when I told them they were perfect just the way they were. A few weeks later, I was surprised to find myself having a good time.

I was in the throes of an especially enjoyable self-appreciation session one morning when the phone rang. Beth was fifteen minutes early for our daily debriefing.

"Whacha doing?" she said. I could hear the toilet flush. Maybe we were too close.

"You mean besides working my ass off, running back and forth to the mall to get Andrew stuff to move into his freshman dorm next month, and buying Ben his first year of high school wardrobe? Actually, I'm standing naked in front of a mirror saying nice things to my body."

She gasped, amused and stricken. "What sadist thought that up? Don't tell me it was the Pussycat."

"That's Tiger to you and yes, he did. You know, it's actually working. I feel kinda hot this morning. I'm in the land of self-love."

"Blech. Glad you are. I'm not. I ate the house last night. I feel totally out of control. I actually scarfed an entire bag of chocolate chips instead of baking the cookies I promised for the school fund-raiser. I have no moral center."

I was in no mood for Beth's rant. It was always hard to hear her complain about her fabulous yogini body when she'd always been thinner than I was—even when I was thin. The age-old competitive streak between us stirred, and I didn't want any part of it. It started with our mothers when we were kids and remained part of their routine to this day.

"Look at those asses on our girls," Beth's mother had said recently as they trailed behind us in the mall. "But your daughter knows how to carry her weight."

I could hear my mother choke. "Yes, she does. She doesn't have time to exercise as compulsively as Beth. Pam barely has time to breathe, her job keeps her so busy."

Their stage whispers made my chest tighten. After all this work I'd been doing to feel even a little bit good about myself, the last person I wanted to compete with was Beth. I loved her. I wanted her to be happy. Actually, I didn't want to have anything to do with the female ritual of self-loathing, a rite of belonging handed down from mother to daughter. I was sick of watching women tear into themselves and each other, a staple of reality shows, sitcoms, and big-screen rom-coms. I wanted a role model who could love herself unabashedly. At the same time, I was afraid that if I stopped making my butt the butt of all my jokes, I would be shut out of the club. I wasn't sure how to change the tribal rules. I didn't know if they could be changed, but I made up my mind I was going to try.

I didn't take Beth's chocolate chip bait. Instead, I invited her into my latest plan.

"Listen, honey. I'm signing up for a workshop that the Tiger thinks would be great for me. You should come, too. It'll be a blast."

"Oh, I don't have time for that. I need to go on the open studio walk in Brooklyn next week. I'm looking for some new blood for the gallery. There's this artist who's fantastic. And unbelievably good-looking. Maybe you should come with me."

"I'll come with you if you come with me. C'mon, Beth. 'Celebrating the Body Erotic' isn't until just before Christmas. That should be enough of a heads-up even for you. You can fit it in."

"Pam, really. The Body Erotic? Sounds a little fringy if you ask me," Beth said.

"I'm not asking you. I'm telling you. It's legit. Besides, how can you resist three days devoted to celebrating our relationship to our bodies and our sexuality? You may find the answer to Kevin and the chocolate chips. You can stay at my place and I'll drive us into the city. Ple-e-ease."

I was in selling and she was powerless to resist. She bought in. I didn't tell her about the erotic massage that we were going to learn to do on each other. That could be her happy ending.

Chapter Fourteen

Rockin' It at Babeland

I WAS ON A touch binge and Markus couldn't stop feeding me. Each day my in-box was full of suggestions for more workshops; important articles about diet, health, and sexuality; other practitioners to sample; and, naturally, my horoscope. It always surprised me that he urged me to work with other people. Did he want to get rid of me? Was I too much? Was I wearing him out? Being a woman of big appetites—my mother always said I was "greedy for life"—it worried me. So I asked him.

Markus laughed. "Honey, I love working with you. That's not the point. When you try other practitioners you find out something new about yourself. They're going to bring something different to the table than I do. Listen, Sacred Intimacy—which is what we're doing, doll—is a conversation between two people. We're doing great. But you don't want to talk to only one person forever, do you? I'm suggesting that you speak with your body to different people every once in a while and see what comes up. Do the Body Erotic workshop and you'll see."

When I admitted the truth to myself, I did want to try it all. Over the past few months I'd gone from being a woman at war with her body and self to beginning to like who I was. I wasn't invisible anymore. Men were holding open doors and rushing to pick up my cell phone when it fell out of my purse, which it always did. Their attention thrilled me. It had been forever since I'd felt like an object of desire, not since the hot and heavy early days of my romance with Gavin. Back then, I was young, slim, and a huge flirt. Gavin couldn't get enough of me. These days, we were so accustomed to each other that neither of us could remember the sexual fire that once consumed us. I hadn't even known that I missed it. It turned out that I did. Desperately. When my friends talked about their lovers, I could see how intoxicated they were by being wanted in a bodice-ripper, can't-wait-another-second way. I finally had to admit that I wanted that, too. My dilemma was how to get that rush without breaking my own rules about marriage. Once I got that Markus actually relished working with me, I imagined how exhilarating it might be to have a practitioner who desired me. I wanted to try a straight man or, at the very least, a bisexual one.

I talked about it with Markus over the Labor Day weekend. He mulled it over for a few days before he suggested Rock. "He's an icon in the sacred sexuality community, known for working with thousands of women."

"Thousands? You serious?"

"Oh yes, he's a SI god," Markus said. "Rock teaches other Dakas how to create transformational experiences for their clients through their bodies."

I had no idea what he was talking about. Daka? You're welcome. Another new word for my SAT prep.

"I'm ready for a 'safe, contained transformational experience' with a hetero erotic rock star," I said a little hesitantly.

"It's going to be great, princess. Why don't we discuss this over lunch?"

"I'd love to," I answered, delighted that he wanted to be my friend. This was definitely off the clock and it felt special.

Naturally, I Googled Rock, just to see. Well, hello. He was a chiseled shaman, riveting in a Red Hot Chili Peppers, Anthony Kiedis kind of way. He looked to be about fifty, hard bodied, with sharp planes to his face and straight hair down to his waist. "Daka Rock" scaling the red cliffs of the Southwest. Rock crouching naked behind a strategically placed giant phallus of a cactus. Rock squatting in front of a fire with his face painted, I guessed, for some ancient ritual. Rock swimming. Rock under a waterfall. Rock at the Great Wall. He was bee-you-tee-full.

I called him and left a message. An hour later, I was up to my elbows in ground sirloin, making a meat loaf for dinner, when the phone rang. A deep voice asked for Pamela. He was instantly recognizable.

"That's me," I quavered.

"How may I be of service to you?" Rock asked.

How does one answer that question? I mean really?

I knew exactly what I wanted to say. I wanted to say, "Gee, Rock. I want to be naked with you. I want you to give me the most incredible erotic massage of my life and take me to the heights of ecstasy that have never been known to womankind! I want you to tell me that I'm beautiful, that your desire for me is making you crazy. That you're having trouble with the boundaries of our relationship. That you want more of me than is legal. Is that possible?"

Who was this woman who didn't want to hide anymore, who was throwing off the armor? I didn't recognize her, but I liked her. Her flagrant desire made me smile.

What I said out loud was, "Do you work with women?"

What an ass. My bold inner goddess apparently ducked out for coffee. Perfect timing. Of course Rock worked with women, thousands of them.

Rock chuckled. "Yes, darling, I know all about women."

My knees went weak. In a few minutes I was scheduled to see him on his next trip to New York City. He was coming east in late September to run a Sacred Sexuality Workshop and Retreat for Sacred Intimates (Dakas and Dakinis). I'd be ready for Rock. I'd have three whole months of practicing my own version of Sacred Intimacy under my belt by then.

"And Pamela, you might want to consider flying to New Mexico to join me and an amazing group of people in a Sacred Sexuality retreat at my temple the week before Thanksgiving. It's gorgeous that time of year, not that it's ever anything but gorgeous out here."

Temple, huh? It sounded so sexy. A Sacred Sexuality Retreat. I'd have to preorder the turkey. Maybe cater the whole meal.

Calm down, girl, I told myself. Before I ran up a huge credit-card bill, I'd better talk to Markus. I didn't know if I'd be experienced enough for a sex camp 2,000 miles away.

"Wow, Rock. That's a lovely invitation, but I'll have to check my calendar."

"You do that, Pamela." Rock's voice poured through the line like liquid gold. "I'd love to have you there. I'll e-mail information. It's not for another couple of months. You have plenty of time to arrange your calendar."

I hung up feeling juiced. Thankyouthankyou, Markus. I was ready for a new conversation with this man. It was hard to believe that my body could say any more than it did with the Tiger, but I gave my imagination room to run wild.

Aflame, I plunged my hands back into the chopped meat, folding in bread crumbs and my Southwestern jalapeño fantasies. I was so wicked. Gavin was getting a Rachael Ray 30-minute meal. I was getting Rocked.

I bent to put the loaf in the oven when guilt smacked me upside the head. Good. I wasn't a complete sociopath. Would a mac-and-cheese from scratch, the kind with the crunchy topping, ease my conscience? I pulled out the ingredients knowing full well it wasn't nearly enough. Rock was really expensive. Dinner, even made from scratch, was not.

I racked my brain to think what I could do to give Gavin something special. Maybe it was time to put some of the spice I'd found with Markus into my marriage. But I didn't know how to go about it. Sex hadn't been a problem in our house. When we were feeling adventuresome, Gavin and I picked out porn movies together, got turned on, and made love. Beyond that, what was there to talk about? We had sex and it worked. But tingling with the new sensations Markus had unleashed, I realized it had been a long time between triple-X-rated flicks. It was time to stoke the fire.

I had a brainstorm. I'd invite Gavin to come on what Markus called a "desire tour" of Babeland and show him all the goodies. Maybe I'd unveil the couple-friendly Chippendales Diva vibrator I bought on my last outing there. That might inspire him. I wasn't one hundred percent sure about sharing all the dark desires I'd been hoarding until now. But I wanted to bring my husband into my new world, just a little bit. This felt like a safe way to begin.

So on Saturday afternoon, I asked him if he would like to go downtown.

"We could walk around and have lunch. What do you say, honey?"

A half hour later we were speeding down the West Side Highway, the Hudson River gleaming in the early fall sun, sailboats cutting through the current.

"Pam! Look at that old wooden boat. Now, that's sweet. I'd kill to have one of those."

"Yeah, and I'd kill you if you added one more boat to our collection. There's no room at the beach house. Sell one and you can buy that beauty." I sighed, knowing that I really might see him sailing a boat like that one into our tiny slip. After all, Gavin was a seaman, a graduate of the United States Merchant Marine Academy who had spent the first four years of our marriage out on the ocean. It was an obsession he came by honestly. His grandfather, his father, and his brothers were all addicted to the sea.

"Speaking of fantasies, Gavin, I was wondering is there anything in the bedroom that we don't do that you would like to do—besides me wearing a sailor hat?" I was as subtle as a tanker. "I thought that we could go to this great store and buy some grown-up sex toys."

"A sex shop? Great. Does that mean we can make love with the light on for a change?" Gavin was positively optimistic.

"Oh yeah, babe. Not only with the light on, but I also might come out from under the covers." My fearless goddess was stepping out again.

It might have seemed out of the blue for anyone else, but after twenty-five years with me, Gavin knew to expect the unexpected. He smiled impishly. "If you're coming out from under the damn comforter, then we absolutely should go toy shopping." Then he asked the question I dreaded. "What's got into you? Don't think I haven't noticed."

I looked at him and wondered if Markus was all over my face. I was embarrassed for a second. "I'm just feeling frisky. I want us to play, to enjoy each other. I want to kick things up a notch."

His eyes bored into me. Just when I thought I couldn't take another second, he decided to go with it. "That could be fun. I know you steal those kinky Anne Rice books out of my drawer."

I had forgotten that we shared that little pleasure. I needed to pay more attention to this man.

"Well, I was wondering what you might like to try. What do you think about?" I said. I anted up first, brave sexual pioneer that I'd become. "Sometimes I think about being with two men. I love that idea. It seems so sexy to me. It could be fun to have a threesome with you."

I didn't consider what I was saying. I was so used to saying whatever came into my head with Markus. It just flew out of my mouth and lit Gavin's fuse. He exploded.

"I can't believe that you would want to be with other people! That's swinging! I'm not open to that at all." I hadn't meant to, but I'd sucker punched him. I'd had all these new experiences. Gavin hadn't even taken the first baby step and here I was talking taboo. He was such a traditional guy in so many ways, a man who held the same computer systems job for twenty years, a steady dad and partner. He looked at me as if I'd grown another head. I'd spooked him.

"Look," I said, talking fast, trying to put the genie back in the bottle, "you know I have the most limited sexual experience of anyone you've ever met. I want to broaden my horizons. With you. I want to try new things. With you. I'm just putting it out there for us to talk about—like all couples do."

"No way am I swinging." Gavin wasn't mollified.

"Well, me neither. It was just a fantasy. Not something I really want to do." He began to calm down. "So, Gavin, what do you say. A little shopping? Just for us."

"Yeah, okay, I'm game," he said, still looking pissed off.

We splurged on a parking lot and headed into Babeland. Gavin rallied and walked through the sex portal like he was walking into a marine supply shop. My sailorman was instantly hooked. Gavin went right over to the butt plugs and dildos. Who knew? I had been married to him for forever and I never knew he was an ass man. I guess if he was married to me, he would have to be.

Gavin was very busy talking to one of the Babeland staff members, a lovely, tomboyish-looking woman. She was going through the ins and outs of butt plugs, showing him books on anal sex and, oh my, showing him strap-ons. Whose ass was he talking about here? He listened to her pitch as though she were the Rosetta Stone of sex.

I walked over to him and held up a strap-on against my body. "Gavin, what do you think of this one?" He laughed, put it down on a shelf, and instead tossed a beginner butt plug and lube into our rapidly filling shopping basket. I had never seen Gavin spend money so fast in my life. He bought an array of vibrators, some porn featuring bondage and butt play, and nipple clamps. I tossed in a book on the fine art of fellatio; he countered with one on cunnilingus.

Gavin was way more sexually open than I had ever known. He just needed encouragement. Before I began my own journey, I wouldn't have known how to ask him about his desires. This new turn was way cool. I could be his Dakini, his guide. Maybe there was juiciness in our future. We left Babeland with bulging bags.

"That young man was so helpful," Gavin said as we departed.

"What young man?" I asked.

"You know, the young man that helped us with all the toys and information."

"Honey! That was a girl. Trust me!"

Gavin looked like he was going to die. "No! Really? I was talking about all of that with a woman?" Gavin's face turned bright red. I pulled my stunned and embarrassed husband into a bar for a drink. We needed to loosen up for the night that lay ahead.

Let's just say that our spirits were willing. My sphincter? Not so much. We managed to ratchet up the temperature in the bedroom.

But after Gavin got through taking my ass by storm, I sent him on an emergency run to the 24-hour pharmacy for all the Preparation H they had in stock. Anal massage was one thing. This was something else entirely. Let me put it this way, my "rosebud" wasn't purring.

Chapter Fifteen

Crazy Fruit Salad

TRIPPING OVER THE empty tubes of hemorrhoid cream that littered the bathroom, I stripped and stepped into the shower. My body didn't know if it was coming or going between Gavin's wild side and Markus's chef's hat. Thank God there was nobody home when I got back after my session. Even after the bath at Markus's studio, I was still a red-stained mess. I reeked of raspberries. Tantric Tiger was stuck on the theme. I was going to be late for the girls, but then again, I had taken to making entrances.

I drove back into Manhattan, all the way downtown, to the Pink Pussycat, which allegedly had the best martinis in the city. The scent of raspberries and the occasional squish between my legs were evidence of the delicious tale I couldn't wait to tell. At last, I had my own lusty stories. The gang was going to love this one.

By the time I got there, they were already three sheets to the wind.

"Sorry, girls. I had to shower—again—to get the raspberry pits out of my pubic hair. You know how they stick."

Four pair of puzzled eyes turned to me. I achieved the impossible. I stunned them into silence. I waited.

"So, are you going to tell us or not," Vicki said.

I told them how Markus took frozen raspberries and turned them into a sex toy.

"There I was on the mat. You know how it goes. He tells me I'm beautiful. I say I'm beautiful."

"Will you get to the good part, please?" Sophia slurred.

"I'm getting there. I was all worked up, like always, panting like I'm going to have a heart attack, and he started dripping raspberry syrup into my mouth."

"Oh, I do like where this is going," Olivia said.

"You have no idea where this is going," I said. "The Tiger took frozen raspberries and started touching me with them. First on my nipples, then on my belly. And then they were on my clit. I think that they could hear me screaming all over midtown Manhattan!

"The feeling of that frozen fruit all over me was amazing. Then I heard the hum of my vibrator. I opened my eyes as Markus laid the vibrator right on me. By the time he was done, it looked like a crime scene. We were both stained completely red. The juice was everywhere. I can't imagine the cleanup! But it didn't seem to matter to him. He was laughing, having a ball, squatting between my legs, with that vibrator shooting raspberries everywhere.

"Between orgasms I told him he was crazy. To which he responded, 'How does a gay man make a women scream in sexual ecstasy? He turns her into a raspberry soufflé!'"

Beth was laughing so hard, she farted. Olivia and Sophia were wiping tears and howling. Vicki gave me kudos: "I bow in your presence. You've now outdone me."

"Oh yeah? You should have seen me walking to the car. I cleaned off at Markus's and I thought I got it all. But every time I took a step, raspberries literally fell out of me. He had actually put them inside of me. Is that bad? Can I get a yeast infection?"

"No, but you might sprout a bush," Vicki said. "Honey, I'm glad you're having so much fun. But really, Pam, I'm starting to worry about you."

I braced myself. Was it possible I was making the free-love diva squirm? What could she possibly have to say to me? She'd always laughed at me for being the family's lone sexual refusenik. I thought she got a kick out of my zany late blooming.

"Pam, I'm not saying what you're doing is wrong," she said. "I just believe that there should never be a fee for sex or whatever you're calling this. Sex isn't a commodity."

"Oh really?" I spat back. "You don't think you commodify sex in your marriage? Of course you do. We all do. Everything's a trade. Nobody gets anything for nothing. Even you got married because free love wasn't free after all."

I didn't mean to fly off the handle. But my big sister could be a bit self-righteous. I calmed myself and explained, "These are all social contracts, Vicki. I just make the boundaries clear for myself. I am not paying for 'sex.' I pay sexual healers to give me access to experiences I've never had before, experiences I didn't even know I wanted or needed. I told you that if I didn't do something to find my sexual self, my marriage would suffer. And I was suffering. Honestly, I pay because I don't want to find another 'someone special' to get what I need 'for free.' Isn't that what most people do—not just men but women, too? Isn't that the road well traveled? I pay so that I don't have to travel away from my marriage. I pay my healers so I don't have to put out. I pay for what I need and nothing more."

Vicki listened while the girls held their breath. They weren't used to the sisters fighting. The silence was interminable.

"I get it, honey," she finally said.

But it took only a minute for Vicki to start in again. "Do you think that you'll stop working with Markus soon? Do you need to continue to do this work? Gavin is waking up. Your marriage is getting better. How about those sex toys and doing it with the lights on? Isn't that a 'transformation'? What more do you need? You've been at this for, what, almost four months?"

My sister didn't get it. Not really. I thought I was so clear about what my work with Markus meant to me, how many old injuries I was finally understanding and repairing. I'd explained how embracing my sexual, sensual side was making me whole in ways that no other therapy had been able to achieve.

I could see that Vicki was genuinely puzzled by my determination to continue. Here I was, a professional advocate with an undeniable track record for getting complex and emotionally touchy ideas across, failing to make the case with my own sister.

Truth was, Vicki wasn't alone in her confusion. Most of my inner circle had been asking about the end point, repeatedly mentioning how long I'd been at it and how expensive it was getting.

I tried again. "To me, my weekly sessions with Markus are like yoga or exercise. I need to keep it up and not get lazy about my commitment to myself. I have so much to explore. Really, Vicki, I'm finally able to tackle the old patterns that have kept me in pain for forty-three years. You know what I've been through. The compulsive overeating, the shrinks, the fucking anxiety. I know this work costs money. But Markus is way more than my therapist. He's becoming my friend. He's been dragging me to every healer he uses. We've been hanging out—sometimes it's lunch, sometimes it's his astrologer, his Chinese numerologist, who, by the way, gave me my own personal ideogram. You know me, I can't keep that professional-slash-personal boundary. I think we breached that border a few weeks ago in the produce section when Markus schlepped me to the supermarket to teach me how to shop for food that's actually good for me and doesn't taste like cardboard. This is way beyond money. And don't think it's romantic, because it is so not. For once, I'm taking care of myself. Because if I don't, I'm not truly allowing myself to be the person that I can be for my family, friends, or anybody else."

I was panting with the exertion.

"I love you," Vicki said. "But I still think you're nuts."

"I know. You all think I'm nuts. So I have an offer to put on the table. How about you try to experience just a little bit of what I'm talking about and see why I'm so into it. There's a workshop coming up in December for women to explore their body issues and sexuality. It's called Celebrating the Body Erotic and it's coordinated by a real PhD, for your information, Vicki. Her name is Corinna and she's brilliant. Markus introduced us over drinks and she's the real deal. It's three days in Manhattan. No travel costs. No tigers. Beth's already agreed to go. Who else?"

Beth shot daggers at me. Sophia immediately said, "I'm in."

Olivia mumbled an excuse and Vicki said, "Honey, you can tell me all about it."

Chapter Sixteen

Between Rock and My G-Spot

I WOULD HAVE A whole lot more to tell Vicki about than the Body Erotic workshop. My new "hobby" was taking up more time than I ever imagined. Finding out about myself was heady and liberating. This went way beyond my sex quest. It was as fundamental as finding out that I could let calls go to voice mail and the world wouldn't stop turning. I could return the calls to reporters, staff members, and even my beloved husband and children without causing calamity. Turned out, my constant vigilance caused me unnecessary anxiety. It was such a relief to let it go. This was as huge for me as getting naked in front of the mirror.

I was learning the difference between taking care of myself and self-indulgence.

Taking care of myself was my plan for three hours this evening. All I needed to do was figure out what to wear. I'd anticipated seeing Rock for weeks and now it was time. I was like a cat on a hot tin roof. I double-checked the hotel room reservation half a dozen times. I'd been upgraded! I'd racked up so many points traveling to work meetings that hotel management rewarded me with a suite, complete with complimentary champagne and chocolate-dipped strawberries. This could only be a good portent. I was calming a little, bustling about the kitchen, getting dinner ready. The Rock session started at 6, so I didn't plan to be home in time to serve it. Leave it to Ben to drop the bomb.

"Hey, Mom, parent-teacher meetings start at four. Don't forget," my youngest said casually on his way to school.

"For chrissakes, Ben. When were you planning to tell me? After they were over?"

Laughing, Ben said, "Why, you got something better to do today?" and walked out the door.

For the life of me, I didn't know how to pull it off. The only bright spot was that Ben's school was a mere twenty blocks from the hotel. I could squeeze it all in if I turned these conferences into a speed-dating experience. Which is what I did, to the palpable relief of the teachers, who all had the same thing to say: "Ben's extremely bright, but he doesn't apply himself."

I could have just replayed the meetings from last year.

"Ben could be an honors student if he just did the homework," his frustrated history teacher moaned.

"Can't he get extra credit for restoring three bikes and selling them on Craigslist? He made $600. Doesn't that count for something?" I countered.

"Yes, it does," his teacher said, laughing. "Just not here. He still needs to do the assignments. But he's got a bright future."

Yes, he does, as long as I don't tell Gavin. Otherwise Ben would have no future at all. Another report card I'd have to hide or Ben would lose *World of Warcraft* rights. Fine, I'm an enabler. But he is so smart. And Gavin would be so mad. I didn't have the strength.

"I'll make sure that Ben steps up," I said, resolved once again to do what I could to control my son's relationship with school.

I fled the building and drove with my fingers crossed, willing the traffic to part. My tires screeched into the hotel parking lot at 5:23. I raced through check-in and tried to compose myself on the elevator ride to the tenth floor. I made it into the suite in time to empty my bladder, splash water on my pits, wipe the shine from my forehead, and fluff my hair. I had a few minutes to check out the room. It was an aphrodisiac. Low lights, plush sofa, thick curtains, and an enormous bed. The charge of waiting for Rock to arrive gave me goose bumps. Everything conspired to make me feel naughty and more sophisticated than I'd ever felt. Hearing a simple knock and opening the door was one of the sexiest experiences of my life, surpassed only by seeing Rock in the flesh, a seductive smile etched on his bronze face.

"Hello, Pam," he said, and immediately took command of the room and me.

Three hours later I staggered into the hotel bar. Olivia's expectant smile faded when she saw the tears running down my face. "Oh, Olivia, it was nothing like I had imagined. Nothing. I don't know what it was."

Olivia ordered two double martinis and sat quietly, waiting for me to let it out. I told her everything.

Rock took my breath away when he walked in the door. His pictures didn't lie. With thick black hair to his waist, an angular face, and an air of ancient mystical power, he was what I'd been fantasizing about. He took me through the usual preliminaries about boundaries, expectations, and intentions for my session. Rock used now-familiar language and was loving and attentive. He sat close to me on the living-room sofa, his jeans-clad leg brushing against my own soft thigh. I succumbed to his warmth.

He listened to my story and thought for a moment. "I want to do ritual touch with you. Would you be open to that?" I told him I was and asked him to explain.

The G-spot was the Goddess Spot, Rock explained. "In order to have a 'mature' orgasm, to really open up as a woman, you need to explore the G-spot. Would you allow me to do that for you?"

I had heard of the G-spot, but I was always way more interested in my clit than my vagina. But the shaman was on a mission and who was I to stand in his way?

He instructed me to empty my bladder and get undressed while he stripped down. He pulled down the bedcovers and laid towels over the sheets. "I have a feeling you're going to be juicy." Oh God. He warned me that I might feel like I needed to pee when he touched my special spot but that it would pass.

The problem was, I didn't feel sexy or warmed up. I felt like I was about to go under some kind of gynecological procedure, only with a naked wild man.

If Markus taught me anything, it was to ask for what I needed. Knowing what to do didn't make the request any easier. "Rock? Excuse me. But I think I need you to make me feel aroused before you do this." Boy, was that hard to say!

Rock let his hands roam around my body. I started to relax and feel more sensuous. He blew Oms into my belly and they vibrated into my core. His hair got wilder. He looked like he was from another dimension. He spoke a blessing about Mother Earth and invited the wind, the water, or something like that, into our space, to help guide the Ritual of the Goddess. It was like being offered up in a ritual sacrifice. It was surreal.

Rock turned me on my back and knelt between my legs. He slowly entered my core with his fingers and started rapidly thrusting them upward over and over again. This was way too intense. It made me want to pee. I made him stop and went to the bathroom. I had to do this four times before I got used to it! Each time, I begged, "Stop the ritual! Stop the ritual! I really have to go to the bathroom!" And each time, he urged me to hold tight. I couldn't.

Rock was patient. The minute I got back into bed he went right at it again, fast and hard. This was new and strange. It felt violent. My body shifted and a new kind of orgasm built, then released, unleashing a tsunami of sadness. Tears flowed. I didn't know where this wall of sorrow came from. I only know it felt atavistic, from a time before words.

Rock held me while I cried, spooning his body around mine. I relaxed into him, but I was shaken.

My voice trailed off and Olivia said, "How are you doing now?"

"I really don't know," I answered. "I feel like something was ripped from me. It was totally unexpected. The orgasm wasn't at all pleasurable. It was wrapped up in tears, pain, and fear that came from nowhere. Well, nowhere I knew. Whatever these emotions were, they came to life so suddenly that I didn't know what hit me."

"You're not telling me he raped you, are you?" Olivia asked, her brows knitted together in worry.

"No, this was all consensual. I completely agreed to everything. It was just not what I thought."

Olivia began to pepper me with her TV-producer questions, her small hands flying in emphasis and practically knocking off her glasses. She went at it as if getting more information was the equivalent of getting answers. I didn't have any for her.

"I didn't know that kind of pain lived in my belly," I said, stanching the flood of queries. "You know, O, I've felt many things in my sessions with Markus—disappointment, joy, humor, sexiness, and power. This is the first time I feel loss, as deep and old as the hills. I just wish I'd been better prepared."

Chapter Seventeen

Here's to You, Mrs. Robinson

I WAS DESPERATE TO purge the grief that engulfed me after Rock. I was sure nothing could snap me out of it quite like an uncomplicated erotic massage. Not that I had found one yet. I loved Markus, but he sure wasn't uncomplicated. The last thing I needed to do was "process." That could wait a bit. I wanted junk food.

I went to the only place I knew to shop for what I wanted, MassageM4M. Lo and behold, up came "Hot Young Hands." He looked like the perfect bag of chips.

He had pictures of himself under waterfalls and smiling gently into the camera. My goodness, he did look young. But he used the right words: "Sacred Intimacy," "Body Electric," "Tantra," and "breath work." I took a chance and e-mailed.

In a few days, David wrote back.

I've wanted to expand my practice to women for a long time. I have been using sacred erotic healing touch on men for four years and have never worked on a woman. It feels like now is the time. I've been waiting for you.

I loved that he was waiting for me. I was his object of desire. I did everything I could to cultivate that feeling. I bought my first lacy thongs. After a lifetime spent in tummy-control granny panties, I was delighted to find thongs came in my size. The minute I slipped into one, I exuded a sensuality that drew people to me. Apparently, Hot Young Hands could feel my heat right through the ether.

We talked on the phone the following day. It turned out he knew Markus and Rock. It was like everyone in this community was separated by six degrees of Sacred Intimacy, and there was safety in that. I told David we were on. There'd be no deep life lessons, no talk, and no rituals this time. Just fun. I hung a Do Not Disturb sign on my G-spot and got ready to play. I was ready for the laying on of Hot Young Hands.

David's studio was about ten minutes away from my apartment, a thin veil of silk separating my worlds. I parked on the quiet residential street while Orthodox Jewish children played stickball during recess.

David opened the door with a white toothy smile. "Welcome. I'm so glad that you came."

I almost dropped dead. David was really, really young. From his Web site photo, I thought he was in his early thirties. But in person, he didn't look a day over twenty-five. I had just become Mrs. Robinson!

David had big blue eyes, longish blond hair, and a slim, well-toned body wrapped in shorts and a T-shirt. He offered me a glass of water and stepped out of the room, still chattering, so I could disrobe.

"I'm really happy you're here. I could learn so much from you." His enthusiasm made me feel oddly cherished. I was somebody else's miracle. And then it came again, my number one, favorite question.

"Does your husband know you're doing this?"

I rolled my eyes. "No. Not yet." I let it hang until I heard him shuffle and clear his throat. "Well, that's okay. Let's get you to the table."

Now we were talking.

David put on music and came back in. His shirt was off, his shorts were still on. His powerful hands began to give me a lovely full-body massage as he worked his breath with mine. It was a familiar ritual that triggered a Pavlovian response of quiet sensuality.

That lasted for about a minute. "Wow," David exclaimed, "you are so beautiful! I love touching you."

I emerged from my stupor. "That's wonderful, David." I sounded like Anne Bancroft in *The Graduate.* I cracked myself up. David was so excited, he was like a kid in Toys "R" Us, playing with all the knobs and handles. It wasn't what I had signed on for, but I was thoroughly enjoying his unbridled enthusiasm. Well, I wanted to be the object of desire.

Out of my half-open eyes, I watched him remove his shorts. I had a "what's he doing?" moment, which quickly disappeared when he burst out, "I rarely get naked with the men. I don't feel safe enough. I feel safe with you and I want to be naked with you."

The weird thing is, instead of freaking out I felt touched by this young man's trust. How odd for me to be the teacher, the elder, the person making it safe, instead of the other way around.

David's eagerness to explore my body was sexy. It was the first time that I felt like I wasn't the innocent one. I knew something David didn't know. I knew about my body and I knew about women. It was powerful. David asked me to turn over. He took the towel away.

"You are like a goddess! Your body reminds me of the paintings of goddesses that you see in Rome."

I signed contentedly. "I know."

It was as if he was drunk on me, and I reveled in it. I gave him a geography lesson of my body.

"Oh, goddess, I love this!" David almost shouted, moving in with total joy and abandon. "Do other women get this wet?"

"I don't know," I gasped between sensations. "I haven't been with other women!"

It was incredible to me that this young gay man was devouring me with his hands, loving my imperfectly perfect body. I didn't feel overweight or over forty. I felt beautiful and radiant.

"Look! I have an erection!" David announced. "I can't believe how exciting this is! Your body was meant for this. You must have been a high priestess in another life!"

That's me. A reincarnated high priestess of sex.

As we wound down the session, beautiful David climbed onto the table and lay on top of me, resting his head on my breasts. I stroked his hair and touched his back. I looked into his eyes and we held each other for a little while. There was the sweetness of discovery. In that moment, I realized that Rock, the vaunted straight Daka, didn't do for my self-esteem what unpretentious David did.

"Thank you for sharing yourself with me today, David," I whispered.

"No, goddess. Thank you. I think that I healed something inside of myself today. I have been wanting this and you made it safe."

I got dressed and bounced out of his tiny apartment. I heard myself humming, "Here's to you, Mrs. Robinson. Heaven holds a place for those who pray . . . hey hey hey. . . . "

Chapter Eighteen

A Ripe Piece of Melon

I WAS FEELING LIKE a ripe piece of melon with juice and seeds spilling all over the kitchen counter. The kind of summer melon that needs an endless supply of napkins. Rock's Goddess G-spot ritual seemed to have released clogged energy. Opened my chakras or let me cry out some old crap. I was so New Age. Whatever. I felt much better.

I was beginning to believe in my right to have pleasure, all kinds of pleasure. I was always the one baking the cookies for everybody else, and now it felt as though the universe was baking the cookies for me. Not just baking them but telling me in so many ways that I was worthy of them, that I should enjoy them. By putting the cookies into my own mouth, by feeding myself, I was recognizing my own self-worth.

For me, it was always about food.

When I sashayed into the steak house for a lunch date with Bitsy, the maître d' tripped all over himself. He took my coat and pulled out my chair. Maybe he knew I was wearing black lace panties. All Bitsy could do was stare.

"Well, look at you!" she said, entertained and genuinely jealous.

"And look at you. You're wearing lipstick. You look great, Bits," I answered honestly.

"Well, I'm not," she snapped. "The estate lawyer went over Howard's financials with me. I called the accountant and got all the old credit-card statements. That fucking bastard had lovers up the wazoo. He bought his bimbos expensive lingerie for their nights in fancy hotels. Now what am I supposed to do? I can't even take a hit out on that creep. Even when he's dead, he makes me feel like garbage."

Bitsy swiped at the tears and her running nose, smudging her lipstick in the process. I moved my chair close to her and cleaned her face with my napkin.

"Honey, I'm so sorry," I said. "Howard was a grade A son of a bitch ever since I can remember. He just wasn't a nice man. You deserve better. And you need to start taking better care of yourself."

"Like you've been doing? Don't think I haven't noticed. You've been completely unavailable to me. It's been ages since we've even taken a walk together."

The waiter, refreshingly old-fashioned with a white apron and minimal tableside chatter, launched into the specials. We dispatched him with two identical orders for rib eyes, salad, and wine. Bitsy was right; I'd been unintentionally scarce in our friendship of late.

"What I've been doing is a little unusual, Bits. And I wasn't sure if you'd understand, let alone approve."

I decided to tell. Maybe it would help her. "I've been going for special massages."

"Yes, I know. Ricky. He's very nice," she jumped in.

"No. Not Ricky. I've been seeing these male massage therapists who give full-body touch, and it's been transforming."

She looked totally confused. "You mean like in *Sex and the City* when one of those girls went for a happy ending massage? Like that?"

"Yes. And no. I mean, sometimes I have an orgasm, but that's not the point. I thought it was, in the beginning. But it's not. You might have a hard time understanding this, but it's been profoundly spiritual for me. I'm healing body issues I thought would be with me forever."

The food arrived, giving me a couple of minutes to rummage through my head for the right words to explain what I experienced on the table.

When we were alone, I launched in again. "Bits, I had been feeling an untapped desire that had been simmering for years just below my skin. Like my spirit simply bounced around without a place to land.

"For me, the Sacred Intimate's massage table is an altar, a holy place," I told her between bites. "It's where I'm held with kindness and love. I get to see myself through the trained hands of another who has no expectations of me. It's freeing, Bits.

"It's a place of tenderness. It can also be a haven for my passion, anger, or sadness, laughter or simply stillness. It has become my confessional and a place of rebirth. It's all happened for me on the table, Bitsy." I took a sip of water and said, "It can be that for you, too."

Bitsy pushed her plate away. "I'm glad for you, Pam. I really am. But the thought of getting naked on the table for any man is just too much. My libido has been dead for years." She surprised me. There was absolutely no judgment.

"Maybe that's why you're having such a hard time dating. You need to rekindle the flame inside yourself before you look outside. This is work I've been doing. It takes a lot of courage to show up week after week. But I promise you it's worth it. You should at least consider it. I'll introduce you to Markus, my therapist. You'll love him. It's completely safe. I'll even take you there and pick you up when it's over."

She surprised me again. "I'll think about it. Does he have a Web site? And I want dessert."

"Great. They have fabulous red velvet cake here. We can split a piece."

"No way. I want this all for myself."

Now that I got.

Chapter Nineteen

Fantasies Unveiled

Two pieces of red velvet cake later, I was heading to the Tiger for my weekly session.

"So tell me about it," Markus pressed. I really hated the chairs. I couldn't get to the massage table or the mat without first sitting in those stupid chairs.

"Come on, Pam. What do you think about when you self-pleasure? It is great that you are reuniting with the music, but when the music is not working for you, what do you think about?"

Markus's greenish eyes were staring intently into mine. He reached down and rubbed one of my feet. I knew this trick! And like a pathetic puppy getting her belly rubbed, I gave in. "Well, oh God . . . I can't."

"Yes you can. It's just me here. No reporters."

"I really don't want to talk about this!" I averted my eyes and talked to the plant behind his head. "Okay. I like spanking." I waited for the earth to open and swallow me. Nothing happened.

"Does your husband spank you?" Markus wanted to know.

He was so casual, as if he was asking me if I wanted cream or sugar in coffee.

"No! Of course not! I would die! I could never let him do that," I stammered.

"What do you like about the idea of spanking? Can you talk about that?"

Didn't this man ever let up? What did he want? I had already shared my deep, dark fetish. Now leave me alone! Take me to the table.

What I said was, "I don't know. I just like the idea of it, the scene of it all turns me on. The over the knee, little-girl drama of it. The lowered panties."

Yep. I am going to die. Right here. Right now.

"Ah," Markus said, "you like the feeling of surrendering, of being taken." Amazing how that language blunted the embarrassment even though the blood still rushed to my face.

"Yeah, I guess so. . . . "

"So, Pamela, is your intention for this session to feel surrender? How would you feel if I spanked you in session today?"

Like a belly turned to jelly. That's how I would feel.

The energy in the studio had shifted, and it made me nervous. Markus was testing the waters. He was trying to get me to touch my desires. Markus led me to the mat and I saw something that I had never noticed before. Peeking out from under the mat were wrist and ankle cuffs. They were leather with soft lamb's wool lining them.

"Pamela, it is my understanding that your intention for your session today is to experience surrender," he said. Markus was always in the habit of speaking out loud the session's intention.

"First," he continued, "you are going to learn the rules of the road. You are 'the bottom.' I am 'the top.' That means I am in charge. Do you understand?"

I must have nodded because he went on.

"Good. During this session you will feel some deep sensations. Don't think of it as pain or discomfort."

Pain? Right about now, any normal person would go running from the apartment, naked or not. What if he was really a Ted Bundy, one of those handsome, mild-mannered serial killers who'd make dog meat out of me once he got me cuffed? But I didn't run. I never claimed to be normal.

"Pain, that's just perception. I would like you to think about the various kinds of touch that you will experience today as 'sensation.' If the sensation gets too deep for you, you can say 'yellow' and I will slow down. 'Red' means stop. 'Green' means keep going. You can also say nothing at all. But until you say 'yellow' or 'red,' I will continue the game. Do you understand? No other words matter."

I nodded.

Markus gathered me close to him, looked into my eyes, and asked, "Do you trust me?"

I stared back. He had been my teacher for close to six months. He had massaged every part of my body. He had sung to me and fed me raspberries. He had even turned me into a raspberry soufflé! I knew this man.

"Yes, I trust you. I'm just a little scared."

"That's good. Now, turn around." Markus's voice got very deep.

I lay on my back and he fixed the cuffs around my wrists and my ankles. I must have looked like a girl in a porn flick, only this was me. Markus was moving swiftly and surely while he instructed me on how to be a good "bottom."

"Good bottoms do not fight the top. If you want the play to stop, you say 'red.' Remember the words. Good bottoms receive. Good bottoms allow themselves to surrender. Do you think that you can be a good bottom, Pamela? Are you ready to surrender?"

I was trying not to faint. My heart was trying to climb out of my chest. Then the world went dark. A blindfold covered my eyes.

I gently tested the cuffs. They were real. I was pinned. I was going to trust. I was going to surrender. I was going to be sick.

No! I was going to do this right. I was going to meet my fantasy head-on. My work with Markus had built up to this day. It was his deep knowledge of me and what I truly needed in my soul that was bringing me to this place.

Markus pumped up the music and began to touch me softly. It was a seduction. He ran his fingers over the length of me. He talked to me like I was a spooked horse. "What a good girl you are," he said. "You're being so brave."

I was relaxing deeper as his hands worked the muscles of my legs and arms. It was a lovely massage, just enough off the beaten path to be exciting.

Then I felt something heavy, with lots of strands, land with a soft thump on my stomach. He ran it down my thighs and calves. That felt great. What was that? It came again and again, down the length of me. He teased my private places as he went. Oh God! I told myself to breathe. It felt so, so good! He picked up the pace and the thumping got a bit deeper. Oh. Oh. Oh. I knew what it was. Leather!

Markus was softly flogging me. This wasn't painful at all. It was soft and insistent. It was teasing and erotic. It felt so damn good I started to moan with pleasure.

"I see that you like that. That's good." Markus spoke with force. His voice had a force to it—the geisha had given way to the gladiator. It was a high-voltage charge.

His little game of thump and drag intensified to a thwack and a thud, while his other hand worked my flesh. It was so intense I had to breathe like I was in a Lamaze class. Markus encouraged me to keep it up and add in deep sounds. I did. I growled. I moaned. I groaned and hissed and grunted. I was the entire Bronx Zoo. I was getting lost in my breath and my animal sounds. He kneaded my legs, reaching under me to my bottom. I felt like a beast completely lost in sensation.

When I thought I couldn't take any more, he uncuffed me and arranged my trembling body over his lap.

To me, there was nothing as intimate as this. I was naked, exposed, hot and bothered, his flesh against mine. I usually didn't get to feel that. I knew what was coming. I was exhilarated and embarrassed at the same time. Markus was gently stroking my body with—what was that? Definitely his hand, but it was sheathed in leather. He was talking softly, telling me over and over what a good bottom I was being. How brave I had been. His hands still played with all of me, making me sigh and gasp.

"Do you remember the words, Pamela? Red to stop. Yellow to slow down. You can say green for more or just surrender into the more."

And so it began. I felt Markus's leather-gloved hand land on my bottom. It didn't sting at first. The spanks landed on me like the thump of the flogger in the beginning. I gasped. The hand landed again and again. My body stretched out more across his lap as I absorbed the spanking sensations into my body. I felt my legs start to kick a little as he deepened the spanking.

The heat of him, the closeness of him. The position I was in demanded that I give up everything—my pride and my illusions of control. I let go, even if it was just for a little while. I let my body be in this place of deep intimacy with Markus. I absorbed the spankings and my sounds grew louder. My legs kicked harder and my hands reached for something to hold on to. I was in my own dance of surrender and resistance. It was kind of like my life. The spanking was a metaphor for my very existence.

I felt such profound relief as I relinquished control and lost my inhibitions that the tears came. It was not humiliation. Some embarrassment at times, but I never felt small or belittled. I felt like I was being held by a force big enough and strong enough to contain all of me. It was a catharsis. I have never in my life believed that any one could hold all my energy. No one was powerful enough for me to truly surrender to. And here I was allowing myself that experience.

My voice rose from somewhere. "Red . . . please . . . *red, red,* please!" Markus stopped instantly. He gently touched my scorched bottom. That felt so good. The tingling was everywhere.

Markus carefully lifted me from his lap. That separation was hard. I wanted to just lie there with him stroking me softly forever.

Markus told me to rest. I floated in my body for what seemed like a very long time. I felt light, like an old weight had been lifted from my chest. I didn't know what it was, but it was wonderful to be free of it.

Markus played a lullaby. He removed my blindfold and held out a cup of our usual jasmine green tea.

Markus, my jungle boy–geisha, was back.

The session was almost over, but I wasn't ready for the real world yet. I was too open and unsure to get dressed and drive home. I needed a little more time to absorb what had happened.

This was not just a fantasy lived. This was not merely sexual thrills. This was a visceral experience. Something inside me let go and I didn't even know I'd been holding on for dear life. I relinquished control and the world didn't fall apart. I allowed myself to have the desire that I had buried under a mountain of shame, and I didn't die of it. As important, I spent ninety minutes unable to give the past or the future a single second of thought. The power of sensation forced me into the present. Only the moment mattered, and it was freeing.

I asked Markus in a soft voice full of "please don't say no" if he would hold me for a little while. His hands brushed my hair off my face as he enfolded me in his arms and rocked me gently.

I don't remember the drive home. I walked into my house after the session, about an hour after I said I would. This was the first time that I was sure that my adventure was as visible as a neon billboard. How could it not be? I wondered if my bottom was red. I would have to be careful getting undressed tonight in front of my husband. How could Gavin not see that I was changed?

"Hi, honey. You're late. Everything good?" Gavin was seated on the couch in his half-work, half-home state of undress: khaki pants and an undershirt. As always, his laptop was open and he was typing away.

"Yeah, honey, everything is good. Sorry, I should have called," I answered before heading to the bedroom to change in private.

Gavin is such a good man. I wondered what he would think if he knew that his wife just had a life-altering experience across the lap of another man? Would he leave me? Would he understand that this was not about our marriage? Could he understand that I didn't feel like I was cheating on him? That my journey was something that I had to do to stay married? I knew that if someone wanted to look at my activities through a Fox News lens, I could be branded with a scarlet letter.

I wanted to talk to him and share my experiences. Was there a way beyond "lights on and blankets off" for me to include Gavin? I just didn't know.

So I went to the kitchen and did what I always do. I started dinner.

Chapter Twenty

Okay! I Admit It! I Shop at Chico's

HALFWAY THROUGH MAKING my signature stuffed Cornish game hens with wild rice and pineapple (a one-hour recipe I learned at my mother's hip, perfect for last-minute Passover Seders and post-spanking dinners), Olivia called.

"How would you like to be a sex goddess and get paid for a change?"

"Hi, Olivia. I'm fine, and how are you?"

"Good, good. I only have a minute. I have a proposition for you. You're always making fun of my focus group opportunities, but you can make a quick six hundred bucks for your opinions on female desire and chocolate. You'd be perfect for this. Who knows more about desire and chocolate than you?"

With my buns still burning, I wasn't sure I wanted to focus on desire at this moment. On the other hand, $600 would cover a couple of very hot sessions. Who was I kidding? I was all about desire.

"Intriguing," I said. "What do I have to do?"

"Nothing. Just give them your thoughts. I pitched you as a sex goddess from Riverdale. You don't even have to give them your name or anything about yourself other than that you're a reproductive rights advocate. It's ideal."

"Really? A sex goddess. I love that. Can I be Kate, the Riverdale Goddess?"

"Sure. Why not?" Olivia said.

She'd been making money hand over fist for years doing focus groups. Why shouldn't I? I liked the shiver of daring that came with creating a new persona and unveiling it in public. People were going to be listening to me, seeing me in a way I'd never been seen before. All this and money, too?

"I'm in. When is it?"

"Tomorrow at five. I know it's short notice, but these things always are." Olivia gave me the address before she rang off. I took my hens out of the oven and threw together a salad. I told Gavin and the boys five minutes to dinner. I was used to being interviewed and speaking in front of groups. It was part of my job that I was good at. I loved an audience. Tomorrow's audience, though, would get the sensuous, sexually outspoken Riverdale Goddess. The anticipation was delicious. I knew I was on the cusp of something enormous. I'd been coming out to myself over these past few months; now all of me would emerge from the shadows. Yes, the name was Kate, but it would be pure Pam. I felt the heat of the Tiger's ministrations to my backside and smiled.

By the time I showed up for the focus group, I was feeling every inch the Riverdale Goddess. I had tossed a flowing turquoise cashmere cape over figure-forgiving black pants. Gypsy-queen earrings and smoky kohl-rimmed eyes made the goddess pop. After my preinterview with the focus group coordinator, Gloria, to qualify as the desire maven (clearly I passed with flying colors—oh, how they wanted me), I arranged to maintain my anonymity with the group leaders. It only added to my mystique. I was digging it. Gloria gave me her private number so she could personally escort me to the proper office. That way I didn't have to sign in at the security desk and show my identification. No bread crumbs leading back to this girl. Not anywhere, not any time. We took the elevator to the big agency in the sky.

"Rob, *this* is Kate!" Rob looked at me and smiled a slightly embarrassed, knowing smile. And he did know a few secrets, but certainly not all of them. There are ways in which I'm discreet. Don't laugh. I am.

Meantime, I was dying under his gaze.

"Hi, Kate, I'm sitting here reading your preinterview notes. My, my." Rob snickered.

What in God's name was I thinking? I wondered what exactly he was sweating over as he turned back to the screen. "You know, Kate, now I'm worried about my wife at home. I don't know about all this."

I hadn't been in the office for five minutes and already I was feeling like a bad influence.

Gloria handed me a name tag, which I dutifully pinned to my chest before meeting up with the other participants in a lush setting of comfy chairs, couches, and an extravagant spread of food. There were about six of us volunteers facing at least ten researchers and a videographer. So far, it was fun.

I had my first one-minute existential crisis in the middle of introductions. How was I supposed to announce myself? Am I just "Kate, the Riverdale Goddess"? Do I hint that I have a mainstream life? That on my way down here, I was negotiating to get Larry King to be the master of ceremonies at my organization's annual fund-raiser at the Waldorf Astoria? I was a living sitcom!

We went around the room giving credentials. There were academics, people with big titles at upper-crust department stores and boutiques, fashionistas who ran style Web sites, and jewelry designers. In the middle of this thin and coiffed crowd, there was me—the big midlife sexpot sitting there with no identity other than Kate, doyenne of desire. My mother would be so proud!

When it was my turn, my ego just got in the way. I had to throw in that I did have another identity, that Kate was only part of who I was. I couldn't help it. It was just too weird simply being the resident goddess.

Not that it mattered. I felt absolutely outrageous anyway. I am what I am, and I talk the way I talk. I'm not into the whole "what is she wearing, who is she doing" celebrity cool thing. There were giggles when I talked. There were a couple of scowls. A couple of the women had taken an obvious dislike to me. One in particular was seething. What did I say to make her glare at me like that? Was everyone else picking up on it? Was I offensive?

Maybe it was my free talk about desire that was so uncomfortable for her. We were there to discuss chocolate. Chocolate is all about desire. Chocolate is not broccoli. It's an indulgence. It's something that we bring into our lives with the pure intention of making ourselves feel good. It can make us feel sexy. It can make us feel like we're having a celebration or savoring a secret.

Chocolate is like sex. We make similar decisions about chocolate as we do about sex. Do we allow it in our lives? Do we reach for it? Do we bite into it? Is it for us or only for other people? Do we feel guilty about it? We were talking my language, and I was fluent.

The manufacturer, who paid for the focus group, was coming out with a new candy. It was directed at women. It wouldn't be a million calories. That's all I needed to know, bro. Sign me up now! We got to taste it. It was like a Kit Kat Bar—crispy and creamy, but richer. When I bit into the candy, I liked how it felt in my mouth. I hadn't had a candy bar in a very long time. Perhaps I was too interested in the candy! I had finished mine. Both pieces. It didn't look as if anyone else had even bothered to taste it. I wondered if I could take some home. I was completely focused on the candy. Give me pleasure and I'm looking to make it last and plotting out how I can have it again.

The conversation was going full speed around me. The whole point of this meeting was to help figure out how to make women desire this candy and then put it in their shopping baskets. Should it be expensive and exclusive or something near the supermarket checkout counter? What made a good brand?

These ladies loved the idea of "exclusivity." The fashionistas were drawing parallels between mass-market candy and mass-market clothing. Up popped Chico's! That perked up my ears. I loved Chico's. I could always find a little piece there to brighten up my closet. I was about to say something positive when one of the style Nazis brought down the hatchet.

"Chico's is totally hideous, so Middle America," she sneered. "A dog wouldn't be caught dead in anything from there."

If you were stuck naked in a mall in Kentucky and the only store was a Chico's, you were better off going to church nude, because all Chico's provided was awful fashion-smashing stuff. I shuffled my feet because I'd almost worn a Chico's jacket that day. Good thing I stuck with Eileen Fisher. I bet this bitch sniffed that I had Chico's bags with their colored ribbons stashed in my closet.

Well, didn't that just suck. Chocolate had to be unattainable to be desirable.

Indulgences. That's what this was all about. What we allow ourselves to have. What was it about indulgence and exclusivity that this group was so attached to? I couldn't figure it out. If we couldn't buy this candy bar, would we really want it more, or would we forget about it? Weren't we told enough in this society that certain things are not for us? That we don't belong? That pleasure is available only for the special people? I don't care about exclusivity. I don't care about belonging to the club.

What I had learned over these past few months was that we are all entitled to reach for what we want. It's so hard to feel entitled to desire. I listened to them calculate how to put this simple pleasure out of reach for ordinary women and it made me furious.

Markus often said to me, "Pamela, how much pleasure can you allow?" I had become a student of pleasure, a budding expert in allowing it, in opening my body to it. Pleasure is not exclusive. It's available in so many forms.

"It seems to me I'm the only one eating the chocolate. Um-ummm. You all should try it before you figure out who deserves it." I turned and looked straight into the camera. "The real problem you're going to have is convincing women it's really fine to have dark chocolate desires and to feed themselves. Good luck. And do you have any extra samples I can take home? These are delish."

How Chico's of me.

Chapter Twenty-One

The Red Shoe Diaries

I decided to go to Daka Rock's erotic-yet-sacred sleepaway camp in New Mexico. Over the weeks since the G-spot awakening with Rock, I got to talk it through with Markus and my newfound friend and Sacred Sexuality mentor, Corinna. They assured me that the hurricane of emotion that G-spot massage unleashed was not uncommon.

"You never know what you're going to get with G-spot work," Corinna said. "It could be a mind-shattering orgasm or an ocean of tears. Sometimes, women feel absolutely nothing. It's all within the normal range."

I forgave Rock and forked over a couple of grand for the retreat. I had a serious cover story to concoct. Stealing five days away under any circumstances would have been a challenge. With Thanksgiving around the corner, the excuse would have to be airtight. Beth was going to a yoga retreat at an ashram in a nearby state. Bingo! I told everyone I'd be taking the beginner courses under Beth's watchful eye. She was just fine with it. I'd covered for her plenty of times.

Gavin received the news with skeptical humor. "Ashram? It's not one of those silent retreats, is it? You won't last five minutes." He knew my limits. I had never, ever even considered putting on a pair of yoga pants. I could barely tolerate touching my toes, let alone find meditative peace in a pretzel backbend. I did have a never-used mat, which I pulled out of the back of the closet as proof of my commitment. I told Gavin it was a whole mind-body weight-loss thing and that I could be quiet if it was absolutely necessary. He shrugged and laughed. As far as the kids were concerned, it was no big deal. Andrew was at his college dorm at least half the time, and Ben was content as long as there was cash in his pocket and take-out menus in the kitchen. One less parental unit badgering him about homework.

A few days later, I was en route to the glorious American Southwest with a relatively clear mind. I was free to concentrate on all the important things, like how I was going to be the fattest girl there and be naked with what I imagined would be a bunch of professionally buffed nudists.

I flew from a classic bundle-up New York late autumn day into a New Mexico inferno. I broke a sweat stepping off the plane. Yeah, yeah, I've heard all about how you hardly feel dry heat because it's dry. Bull! It's hot. I schlepped my two overstuffed suitcases bulging with silk kimonos and flimsy muumuus big enough to double as circus tents to the car rental station, where I got myself a flaming red Mustang. If I was going to act out, I figured it might as well be Oscar-worthy. I loaded up the car and set out for two freak-out hours through the mountains. Beautiful. But after five hours of turbulent flight, driving hairpin turns along sheer drops wasn't working for me. By the time I made it to Rock's driveway, my knuckles were white and my nerves were raw. But it was worth every heart-pounding moment.

The Daka's compound was a Shangri-la, once you got past the suburban wooden fence and beyond the carport, past the mundane green siding on the ranch-style house. Through a gate that shielded the inner sanctum from view, I stepped into a wonderland of fountains, stone gardens, hammocks, and old-fashioned rocking benches. A free-form glass-sculpture reflecting pool stood at the convergence of three streams that flowed from the fountains. My spirit soared. Daka Rock's Magic Kingdom.

I unloaded the Mustang and trekked to the entrance. A sign asked me to remove my shoes. How Zen. I kicked off my boots and knocked on the screen door. A slender, thirtyish bouncy brunette named Lily Rose let me in. She might have worked as Rock's innkeeper, but she didn't have a hotel-management thought in her head. She accompanied me as I lugged all my stuff down the hall, giving me a meandering spiel about the Temple's countless attractions, including a detailed description of the buffet breakfast menu. Once I deposited my conspicuously large valises, Lily Rose resumed the tour. We walked past a lapis lazuli–blue lap pool, bordered by small waterfalls that split the backyard down the middle. The pool flowed into the indoor "spa" wing outfitted with a steam room and sauna.

She gestured to a waist-high pool lined with stone and waited expectantly. I complied. "What's this?"

"Actually, it's the Watsu," she said with a giggle. "It's heated to body temperature and is only for water massage."

That's all I needed to hear. I was infatuated with the breathtaking house and grounds, the red rock New Mexican mountains. How could anyone not love this amazing place?

Lily Rose left me in my room with its king-sized bed and unobstructed view of the pools. "We'll all gather in the dining area in twenty minutes," she said on her way out. I unpacked, which was a serious undertaking given the major Nordstrom damage I had done, buying everything that billowed enough to conceal a small village. I followed the trail of genial voices to the retreat rendezvous. About a dozen men and women lounged in a stunning open space with a giant stone fireplace, open kitchen, couches, and table—all framed by glass walls that let the outside in. I was overwhelmed, acutely conscious that at some point we'd all be naked together. My hyperactive imagination tried to strip my classmates to their bare essentials, but I couldn't get past the middle-American suburban zeitgeist: blue jeans and Southwest gear. Everyone was friendly, warm, kind, and ordinary. But who the hell were they? I had no idea. I wasn't even sure who I was. We talked until I couldn't keep my eyes open. I turned in and crashed into a deep, weirdly dreamless sleep.

I woke up raring to go, laughing at myself for being so nervous because there was no course syllabus. At least after last evening's meet and greet I knew who the three leaders were. There was Rock, of course. I'd try to forgive the bad case of G-spotitis he left me with after our East Coast encounter.

There was DC, a big, powerful presence. He must have been in his late fifties, with salt-and-pepper hair, a gray beard, and Paul Newman blue eyes. I knew he was going to be the heart and soul of the retreat—at least for me. Men and women, we all gravitated to him.

And there was Anastasia. I must not forget Anastasia. I took an instant dislike to her. I'm not saying it was rational, but she felt dark. She had long black hair and exuded the sexuality of a Bollywood star. Exotic and pretty, with a know-it-all attitude that raised my energetic hackles. Perhaps there was a teeny bit of jealousy over her lithe body. Maybe it was the way she bragged about being a "sacred prostitute" trained at an ashram in India. Or how she claimed snakes as her personal totem. I didn't have a totem, but if I did it'd have to be the sockeye salmon swimming upstream to lay eggs and die, or show up in a deli case for forty dollars a pound. Maybe my totem was a lemming—show me the nearest cliff, and off I go. Bottom line, I didn't like sitting next to her.

The rest of the group was surprisingly like me. We ranged from our midthirties to the light side of fifty. There were two divorcées, attractive women with young kids at home: Brooke from Kansas and Lee-Ann from Texas.

Tim and Becky were Tantra teachers from Georgia and had been married for years. They were at the retreat to sort out some marital bumps that popped up from their work. Jill made it from Florida; Heather from Boston; and Richard and Mike from Ohio and Minnesota, respectively. We were a cross section of America, familiar and foreign.

After a light breakfast, we gathered in the workshop room, an enormous white space dotted with white pillows of every size and shape. Only the floor-to-ceiling windows opening on to the pools and cliffs kept me from going snow-blind.

Everyone was clad in blue jeans, sweatpants, tank tops, and T-shirts. No makeup, which made me a standout. I swept into the room in a flowing pink silk muumuu with white flowers and kimono sleeves and coordinating pink lipstick. I was hard to miss, but no one said anything.

"Will you all seat yourselves in a circle? Please take the pillow of your choice. We want you to be as comfortable as possible. And do make sure you have lots of water," DC began. "We don't want anyone getting dehydrated."

Dehydrated? Why would we get dehydrated?

There was a brief flurry of activity while we got ourselves arranged. The circle, I learned, would be the motif of the week.

DC started us off by asking us to say our names and tell a bit about our lives and what we hoped we'd get out of the retreat. Maybe the Temple was built on a mystical vortex or people figured what the hell, but the soul-baring was intense. People's stories ran the gamut from divorce to fear of intimacy to abuse. They talked about their pent-up, misunderstood sexuality, their scary desires, and their pain. Exhausted by the trip and circle talk—it took two hours and two boxes of tissues to get to me—I didn't have the energy to give them much more than the basic body image, weight, and sexual exploration outline. Still, I managed to add my own soaking tissue to the pile before Rock called it time.

"Folks, it's nice and hot, sunny and beautiful," said Rock, the perfect B&B host. "Why don't you enjoy the pools before lunch."

Everybody let out a whoop. Recess! We stampeded the door.

I went into my room to get my bathing suit. I had brought three, each with a different skirt length to correspond with how I felt about my thighs that day. I happened to glance out the window and saw people jumping naked into the water. I was startled. There were jiggling penises and flashes of pubic hair. I caught myself mentally scanning all the bodies to see if I'd be the fattest person in the pool. It was a horse race between me and Heather. She was as zaftig as I was. I was embarrassed by how relieved I was to see cellulite dimpling her body.

Okay, then. No bathing suit. But I wasn't walking across the grass without a cover-up. I opted for another kimono, black silk with brightly colored tropical flowers. I mean, once you get a look that works, you stay with it, right?

Richard, Jill, and Brooke were in the hot tub. I sucked in my breath and casually tossed off my robe. I stepped into the pool. I was relieved to be submerged until I noticed that my breasts were floating on top of the water. Well, that's just great. Miss Tits! How was I going to convince my C-cup girls to get down and stay down? How was I going to manage all this public nudity with this body?

"Pamela, can I tell you something?" Brooke's question brought me out of my mental monologue. I looked over at her. Brooke was beautiful, tall and slim, with perky B-cup breasts. She was perched on the side of the hot tub, dipping her feet and not hiding a thing. Even her pubic hair was coiffed. Oh well.

"Of course you can, Brooke. What's up?" I tried to look into her eyes, away from her boobs.

"Well, I just have to tell you, I mean, I don't want to embarrass you, but you have the most beautiful breasts! I am sitting here feeling so jealous of your breasts!"

My mouth dropped open. "You were admiring my breasts? That's too funny! Brooke, I have been sitting here feeling like a big blob with breasts that are just too much. I've been wanting your breasts!"

And so it began. I was in the land of sacred mirrors. We looked into each other and saw great beauty. What a gift. And all before lunch.

By day three I was feeling confident, maybe a little smug. I had dropped my muumuu; I'd danced naked in a trance with my campmates as we embodied the four elements—fire, earth, water, and wind—on DC's command. I was lost in space when Rock cleared his throat and brought me back with a thud. "For this next exercise, please get a towel and anything you'd like to use to self-pleasure."

I knew what "self-pleasure" meant. I was all over this lingo. Self-pleasure where? In the workshop space? In a group? C'mon. He couldn't be serious. Omigod. Apparently I was the only one having an "oh shit" reaction. The rest of the crew didn't hesitate before scurrying off to gather their "personal" items.

What does one wear to self-pleasure in a circle? I had no idea. I took off my sexy undies and wrapped myself in—what else—a kimono and grabbed a towel. That ought to do it. Wrong. I was dumbstruck by the paraphernalia people trucked in. Two women were recharging their vibrators and exchanging the 411 on dildos. Naturally, the men didn't need much beyond their hands. There was massage oil and lube on a table. I had to rally. I wasn't going to be the lone chicken. I had a vibrator. I could play, too! I ran to my room, breaking out in a rash as I raced back.

We re-formed our circle, trying to get comfortable for God knows what.

Anastasia, she of the ashram, explained that not only were we going to self-pleasure together this morning, but we'd also bear witness for each other. Sure. Of course we would. Anastasia showed us how to breathe up our sexual energy through our loins and into our pelvic floors. She prattled on about how breath and working our muscles could heighten our sexual pleasure while demonstrating the proper way to clench your butt and thrust your hips. Then she walked around, coaching us while we all practiced breathing and clenching.

To add to the merriment, Rock brought out his bag of Magic Wands. These supposedly helped women find their G-spot during any kind of sexual activity. I swear, the man was G-spot obsessed. The wands were made of brightly colored Plexiglas bent into S-shapes with a knob on one end. For about thirty bucks, one could be yours. Gotta give Rock credit, he was quite the pitchman. The ladies closed in. They dug through the big bag, exclaiming over all the different colors and knob shapes. I hustled over. Even though I wasn't exactly friends with my G-spot, I didn't want it to feel shut out. The red ones were going fast. I went for pink. It worked with my outfit. The men watched in bemused wonder while we "shopped."

Once the frenzy subsided, DC got us to settle down. DJ Daka

Rock spun New Age electronica to set the mood. DC instructed us to "get comfortable," which translated to "disrobe" for everybody else. Not me. I hung on to my kimono like it was my first blankie.

Jeez, everyone was so gung ho. I didn't wanna masturbate in a circle. How about a hole in the earth? That would work just fine for me. This was way too intense. I grudgingly made a little nest with my towel, my kimono, and my pillow. I carefully laid out my vibrator and my new pink G-spot wand. And all this time I thought I only needed fingers and the occasional fantasy to get off. Such a naïf.

Before I could say "Hostess Twinkie," a bunch of folks were going at it. I could hear panting, breathing, groaning, and sighing. Me? I felt like the Little Engine That Could. *I think I can, I think I can!* looped over and over in my head to no effect whatsoever.

I cracked open an eye to take a peek. Tim, right there next to me, was in full stroke. Oh. My. God. I shut that eye right up.

"Feel your pleasure. Feel your pleasure. How much pleasure can you allow your body to have?" DC was like an evangelical preacher shouting about the glories as he walked among us checking our progress. "Remember to witness your neighbor's pleasure."

Anastasia was cheerleading, "Breathe, breathe. Clench. Breathe."

Rock was making orgasmic sounds. "Ahhh, yes, oh yes, beautiful."

I looked at Tim again. I'd never seen a man masturbate. It was kinda cool. I turned my head and there was Becky, Tim's wife, on her knees with her fingers working between her legs, one hand on one breast. Her eyes met mine! She saw me watching her husband and then her!

I wanted to disappear. My body went flat against the floor. I gave myself a good talking-to. *Honey,* I told myself, *you better get cracking! Focus!*

I reached down between my thighs and located all my parts.

Anastasia, DC, and Rock continued their walkabout, "holding space," endlessly chanting encouragement.

"Feel your beauty."

"No one is responsible for your pleasure but *you.*"

"You have the power to give yourself joy!"

"Feel the fire in your loins."

"*Breathe!*"

Nope. I didn't think so. Uh-uh. I wasn't turned on. I was having performance anxiety. I knew DC knew that I was flunking self-pleasure. It was embarrassing. I tried to hunker down again. But I was like that girl in *A Chorus Line* when she sang, "I reached right down to the bottom of my soul . . . *and I felt nothing!*"

So I marked the time. I waved my new wand. I breathed and clenched. I played with my pelvic floor muscles. I wondered if it was really insane to fake my own orgasm. It was unbearable.

People were climaxing all over the place, gradually coming "back" from their journeys. DC said quietly that we were now free until after lunch. *Thank God.* I gathered up my toys and escaped to my room. I needed to shower off the morning.

The workshop flew by and I couldn't believe it was almost over. Our fearless leaders, the Three Sex-keteers, were taking us on one last hike into the mountains. I was scared of heights, tunnels, bridges, and things that go bump in the night, so while I loved hiking along straight paths, I was dreading the rocky ascent up the cliffs of New Mexico. I hadn't brought the right footgear. All I had were shiny, red silk, rhinestone-studded Nikes. They were so Dorothy! It's why I bought them. I loved the concept of the ruby slippers. I loved that Dorothy had the power within her to take herself home the whole time she was in Oz. All it took was three clicks of her heels. So I put on my own "ruby slippers" and joined the tribe as we made our way up the mountains.

The hiking was only moderately difficult. I was relieved. I made my way, carefully avoiding the cacti that were everywhere. We scrambled up some rocks, and boy, was it hot. Finally, I could see that Rock was leading us right to the edge of a cliff with a beautiful view way down below. Now I wanted to hurl. I could feel the beginnings of a panic attack coming on. But I was determined to do this. This whole trip was about facing my fears. This was simply another one of them.

When we got to the top, my fellow campers climbed onto a boulder ledge two feet below the lip of the cliff. With the sun against their backs ringing them in a halo, Rock, Anastasia, and DC gave us a talk about Mother Earth, the Four Spirits, and self-discovery. Rock squatted, bare-chested, hair blowing, waving a big eagle feather to make his points. I couldn't concentrate on a thing they were saying because I was glued up against the boulders trying not to vomit. Yeah, sure, I knew the sun was beginning to do the setting thing and it was gorgeous. I just couldn't care less. I kept my eyes mostly closed, trying not to freak out.

After they wrapped up the talk, they encouraged us to spend some time in thought and meditation. They said that no one was around, so if we wanted to feel the sun on our bodies, we could undress. Several folks were already shirtless, laying back and soaking in the last rays and heat.

I kept my eyes shut and began a short meditation focusing on breath. The magnitude of what I was doing, the courage it took for me to get through this week, warmed me like that blazing desert sun. In a second—that's all it was—the Riverdale housewife gave way to Xena, Warrior Princess, and my old myths, the ones that kept me sequestered in muumuus, shattered. I got up from my secure perch on the boulder and walked around the edge of the cliff. It was so beautiful. And with a feeling of rebellion, I began to undress. There I was, the woman with the shame of her body, the woman who needed to lose sixty pounds, the woman who struggled with using food to mask her feelings, the woman who always championed others, finally standing up for herself. I took off every stitch of clothing except for my ruby slippers.

I was naked and strong. I looked out at the endless sky and flat desert and I raised my hands up to the heavens. I felt such power. I let my hands roam over my body. I touched my breasts and my nipples. I let my hands span my belly and run down my ass. I held my vulva in one hand and put the other hand on my heart. I wanted to be with my inner goddess. I wanted to feel her! My God, I was a commanding woman! I felt it and I owned it. I got it fully that we have to stand up for what we want on this earth. Others may very well judge it, condemn it, and laugh at you. This world is not necessarily forgiving. We like to think that if we follow our desires and dreams, those around us will support and love us. But it doesn't always work that way. We have to really be committed to our own truths and be prepared for the occasional shit storm.

I turned around to my group of newfound friends. Some were in their own worlds, but Anastasia was watching me. She smiled.

"Pamela, I wish that I could take a picture of you, you look so beautiful."

I wanted to freeze that moment in my heart forever. It was Anastasia, the woman I couldn't warm up to, who gave me this extraordinary gift. She helped me take my own mental picture: The image of me naked on those rocks, facing my fears about who I was and who I could be, about how high I could climb. Something snapped into place. I was ready to click my heels and come home.

Chapter Twenty-Two

When Worlds Collide

I LANDED BACK IN New York on a high. I sniffed the first damp gusts of winter and took in the blazing white of a fresh, light snowfall. I felt vaguely alien after New Mexico, but exotic and erotically energized. I wanted to rub some of the magic off on Gavin.

When I got to the apartment, the boys gave me a grateful "Thank God."

"Dad never lets up when you're gone," Ben tattled. "He's always nagging about homework or cleaning up."

"Or something. What's for dinner?" Andrew said. "Dad has no clue about grocery shopping. I'd rather starve than eat another grilled cheese sandwich."

"You guys didn't order in? I left money and menus."

The boys shot daggers at me. "Dad said it cost too much and he could cook," Andrew said.

Apparently, my notion of a 24-7 toga party was misplaced. Gavin had overcompensated for my absence. The boys were so happy for the return to normal. They had their Daddy buffer back and the promise of real food. I dropped my bags and hugged them as much as they'd let me.

"I swear, no more American cheese. We'll order Chinese tonight."

Yeah, Dorothy was home. There were dishes in the sink, a turkey to buy, countless messages from my mother reminding me about the side dishes, and my business line blinked furiously. I wasn't going to answer a single message until I had my time with Gavin. I was doing everything I could to hold on to the saucy seductress I wanted to bring home to him. Maybe tonight we would dig into that Babeland bag again and I could show him how flexible I gotten from doing all that "yoga."

Early the next morning, still jet-lagged and feeling the vestiges of the Four Elements, I woke up in time to listen to my messages before getting on a call with Bob. Markus had left a voice mail that he was on his way over to borrow folding chairs for his men-only "empowerment" group. Again. Maybe I should just go to Lowe's, buy him a few, and save him the schlep. The phone rang.

"Pammy, hi, it's Mom."

'"Hi. How're you? What's up?"

"I'm on the cell. I love using it. I never use up my minutes. So listen, I'm right outside your building. I'm on my way to bridge. I'll ring your bell. I'll only stay for a minute. I want to see how that yoga worked. I'm thinking I should take some classes at the club. They finally got with the twenty-first century. The step classes? Bor-r-ring."

"No, wait. Mom! I have a conference call. I can't." I had sudden onset tachycardia. Markus and my mother in my apartment? Shitshitshit.

"A minute, Pammy. I'll be in and out."

Famous last words. Within seconds, the buzzer sounded. I let Mom in and gathered up the folding chairs, ready to thrust them at Markus before he set foot inside.

The elevator door clanged open and Mom was in the door.

"You look wonderful, Pammy. You got color."

I grabbed her arm and pulled her into the kitchen, as far away from the door as our minuscule apartment would allow. "Here, have some coffee. Wait here, I have a present for you."

The buzzer rang again.

"You expecting someone? At this hour of the morning? You don't have the housekeeper today. It's Vicki's day."

That poor housekeeper. She worked for my mother, my sister, and me, and Mom kept tabs. We drove that woman insane.

"No, Mom. Just a friend who needs to borrow some chairs."

Markus knocked. He couldn't have waited ten minutes? I opened the door and there he was, his sandalwood musk punching a hole through the hot coffee aroma.

"Here are the chairs." I didn't give him a chance to say hello. I pushed the chairs into his arms. "Sorry, Markus, I don't have a second. Conference call. Love you."

"Okay, okay. Thanks. Love you, too."

I pecked him on the cheek and shut the door. I turned back into the apartment. Mom was lying in wait, smiling that sly smile that made me a wreck my whole life.

"So who was that? You couldn't invite that handsome, *handsome* man in for a little coffee?"

I gagged and coughed and made up my mind. "That was my life coach. I didn't want to say anything about that just yet."

"You're seeing a life coach? What for? You could *be* a life coach."

"He's more like a personal trainer, Mom. Helping me with food and lifestyle. Things like that. He's very talented."

"I can see that he's doing a good job. I didn't want to say anything because I know how sensitive you are about your weight. But I really see the difference."

I sighed. Even with a compliment, I still felt sized up.

"Okay, I should go. I'm late for bridge. I just needed to see you after a week. I'm bringing the coffee cake, not that I would touch it. I'll call you later."

She disappeared out the door scant minutes after Markus. God, I hope they didn't collide in the street. My life was pure *Seinfeld.*

I barely had time to pee before Bob called to go over my e-mail about expanding our mission to bring sexuality into the fertility field. The science was mounting that healthy sexuality was linked to everything from infertility prevention to divorce prevention.

"Fabulous idea," he drawled. "Now, if y'all can figure out how to bring the possibility of healthy sexuality into my life, I'd underwrite the whole damn program."

"My, my! Not getting much, Bob?" I knew his partner's three kids had recently moved in. The ex-wife had freaked when he announced he was gay after fifteen years of marriage and fled to do her own version of *Eat, Pray, Love.* This was not what Bob had signed on for.

It didn't take much prodding for him to let loose. "Monogamy was hard enough for me. Throw in three angry kids and I'm feeling like I'm ready to jump ship. I don't want to, but. . . . "

Sounded like Bob needed a little Four Elements of his own. Before I could think about what I was going to say, I started to blurt, then stopped.

"Can you keep a secret? I mean you tell absolutely no one."

"Sure. Pinkie swear. Not a problem. What's the big deal here?"

"Bob, I completely understand what you're going through. But

I've been doing a kind of therapy that's giving me heat back in my own life. Maybe you don't have to bail on your family. There's this great guy in New York City who's a Sacred Intimate and does one-way touch. You'd love it. And him. He's gorgeous and he's gay."

Bob pumped me for every detail and I flowed like Niagara Falls. He loved that I was working with a gay man for sexual healing. In that moment, he became my new BFF.

"You know, Pam," he confided, "I've done just about everything when it comes to sex—things that would burn your innocent ears. But I've never done this."

"You should. It'd be good for you."

"Yeah, but I think if I do a session, I'd like to do it with my partner. It might move us to a better place. It's intriguing. It's obviously doing wonders for you."

Chapter Twenty-Three

Fearing the Scarlet Letter

I hung up and made the bed. The pillows still had the imprint of Gavin's head. I felt like a hypocrite. Here I was talking up the benefits of my explorations to my work peeps, and I couldn't tell Gavin. It was absurd and starting to feel dangerous. Not only couldn't I keep my mouth shut, I was a lousy liar. I needed to tell him. I just didn't know how. I closed the apartment door behind me and headed for a day packed with organization meetings.

Everything was back to the way it was, except me. Everyone, even my kids, picked up on how much happier and less cranky I'd been in recent months. It was only Gavin who didn't notice how much I'd changed. How was that possible? It occurred to me that maybe for Gavin things were not that different after all. Our routines were more or less intact. Dinner was on the table every night,I perked coffee for him every morning, and most evenings we sat side by side on the couch with our laptops open and a movie on the TV.

Unexpectedly, the fear that I thought I had left on the New Mexico cliffs reared its head. What would happen when Gavin found out? Would he understand that I simply needed to explore myself in a way that wasn't a part of our marriage bed?

How could I explain to him that what I was experiencing was profoundly different than lovemaking? Lovemaking is about the union of two people. This was about me. It wasn't a two-way street of emotion the way it would be with a lover. Sacred Intimacy and sensual massage showed me how to love myself in a way that I had never thought possible. I was experiencing joy—true joy—in my body.

Driving into Manhattan for the meetings, I found myself making speeches to Gavin and they all sounded tone-deaf. I went into a full-blown anxiety attack, my mind filled with anticipatory doom. What if he condemned my "therapy" as cheating? What if he thought I was a completely mad nympho? And worse, what if he thought I was selfish? My thoughts spiraled from there. What would the rest of my world think?

The hardest part about this route to my self was the fear that if I ever talked about it outside of my closest circle of friends, I could lose everything that I held dear.

There were no precedents in this culture. I hadn't seen this on *Oprah* or even *Howard Stern.* What normal woman did this? I was sure Dr. Phil would have words for me. "What are you thinking?" he'd shout at me while the audience booed and stomped. Oh yes, he would love to get me in one of those high chairs as he exposed my moral misdeeds before all of America. Maybe the ladies on *The View* would be kinder. They're free thinkers, aren't they?

Television was filled with shows about "emotional affairs" and "cheating wives." But I'd never heard one talking head take on the world of Sacred Sexuality or the healing power of sensual touch. No one was revealing how working with sexual healers could actually save a marriage. I knew it was saving mine.

Funny, we as a society have no trouble blabbing endlessly about alleged self-improvement, which usually boils down to getting skinny and trying to stay young. Every TV and radio show featured yet another doctor, actress, or athlete who had found the ultimate weight-loss program. There were people extolling the virtues of cutting up the stomach or binding it to control food cravings. There were infinite broadcasts and podcasts about how plastic surgery could make you into the something better you could never be without it.

But there was nothing about learning to love yourself now, just as you are.

I was gripped by panic that the people outside my world would reduce me to an unfulfilled midlife sex fiend. The only images of women who pay for sexual services were the women who wanted to get their rocks off in *American Gigolo.* Was that me?

Was Markus a gigolo? Absolutely not. He was a healer. Escorts and gigolos do what you want them to do. Markus hardly ever did.

There wasn't any fucking going on between me and Markus. Or anywhere else in the workshops and sessions I went to.

From everything I saw, this wasn't some great big swing party. People were using sexual energy in a way that I had never known it could be used. It was a kind of whole-body therapy to help people integrate their beings. Sexual energy is powerful, hypnotic, and potentially terrifying. Even if it doesn't look the same from person to person, we all feel it when we're in its presence. It rolls off some people, like Bill Clinton, Sophia Loren, Sean Connery, Madonna, or, God help me, Sly Stallone. Sexual energy affects behavior and judgment and has ruined careers or made them. Cleopatra, Henry VIII, and John Edwards invaded my head. Maybe that's why we're so afraid of sexual energy. Maybe that's what I had been afraid of all my life. I spent a lifetime tamping down my own sexual energy and power. Now I was tapping into it. I couldn't fathom explaining this to Gavin.

I knew I had stumbled onto something remarkable, yet no one was talking about it anywhere. My evangelical side was kicking into gear with each new person I felt safe enough to tell. I saw how hungry Bob, Bitsy, and even my adventurous Martini Gang were for any scrap of information that might lead them on their own path of exploration. I wasn't alone in my need to connect to the whole self. They all wanted the same thing.

But I knew how easy it could be for a stranger to plaster me with labels. How would Pam the Advocate ever explain the experience to someone like Dr. Phil?

Never mind Dr. Phil and the rest of the world. The biggest thing for me was right in my own bed. I needed to tell Gavin. Soon.

Chapter Twenty-Four

Goddess in Green Cellophane

I HAD SO MUCH going on inside my head, so much I couldn't explain. I needed to be with someone who understood. I wished it could be Gavin, but it wasn't. Right now, it was Markus. I needed him to help me reconnect to what I had felt in New Mexico, that naked goddess in her ruby slippers. I wanted to feel her again. She was too new; she felt like she was slipping away under the weight of my job, the dishes, and my mother, who was annoyed that I didn't have time to take her to Lord & Taylor to return a bathing suit.

Markus was as impatient for our next meeting as I was. He'd never been to Rock's New Mexico "temple" and wanted the inside skinny. He promised something special if I told him every little thing, his voice sexy and mischievous. The last thing I wanted to do was talk.

I rang his bell, proffering gifts of colored beads and a tiger mug, early Christmas presents. He loved the beads and was almost polite about the mug, which promptly disappeared from sight, never to be seen again.

He made a beeline for the chairs. I piped up, pushing my agenda, "Could we talk later? I really want to go to the mat!"

"Oh? We are in a hurry today. Where's the fire?" he asked. And he gave me such a look that I turned bright red. Markus laughed with his whole body. Apparently I was very amusing.

"Okay, goddess, you want to check in later? We can do that this once, but we will talk about it all . . . okay?"

The screen was up and I couldn't see the futon.

Markus got up, went behind the screen, and was gone for a few minutes. When he came back he was wearing black chaps and a G-string. He had little red devil horns on his head. They peeked out from his hair. He was too hot for words.

"Today, you are going to get your next lesson on being a bottom. I think that you're ready after all of that time in New Mexico!" His eyes were twinkling.

"Do you like my horns, Pamela? You know, they're not something I get to wear very much!" Markus was still having fun with me.

"Now come here. I want you to fasten my leather cuffs on my wrists. A good bottom knows how to do this for her master." Without skipping a beat, I walked over to Markus and laced up the long black leather cuffs as if I'd been doing it forever.

"Good girl. Now I want you to get undressed. Right now." Markus's voice got markedly deeper. It was clear he was now the alpha dog and I was to obey. My stomach started to do its "Oh boy" dance.

While I was stripping, Markus took away the screen. There was a massage table where the futon used to be. Once I was naked, I walked over to the table and leaned my elbows on it.

"Oh, that is a good idea. Bend over the table," he commanded. "Now."

I did as I was told. I bent over at the waist. My upper torso was resting on the head of the massage table. My arms were in front of me and my feet felt sturdy on the ground.

"Okay, Pamela, I am going to tie you today. You remember the words, right? Red to stop. Yellow to slow down. Green or nothing and the game continues."

The temperature was rising fast. Markus handled my body in a very purposeful way. He had a roll of green cellophane wrap. I could hear it tearing as he started to wrap my body. Aha, these were my ropes for the day.

First, Markus pulled my arms out in front of me and bound them to the table. Then he spread my legs in a V so I could feel the air all over. That could make a girl breathless! He was methodically cinching my ankles with the cellophane and fastening me to the sides of the table.

And then the cellophane started to work its way up my body. Markus was building a corset for me out of the stuff. He tightened the plastic around each of my breasts, like a balloon. The feeling made me gasp with mind-boggling intensity. He teased my nipples just for extra enjoyment! *Oh God!* And that boy kept wrapping!

He worked the cellophane down my body and through my legs. He pulled it back and up so that it was strategically riding between my buttocks and the cleft of my vulva. He finished his knot somewhere in the middle of my back.

Markus tested his handiwork by pulling up on the corset between my legs. It was very strategically placed. What a charge!

"Oh, good. I did a great job!" Markus chuckled.

I had a very strong feeling of being held. I liked it.

Next, Markus tightly tied a scarf around my eyes and gave me a very sharp spank on my bottom that was totally unexpected. If I could have jumped ten feet into the air, I would have! A little tape went off in my head, "Lucy! You're in *trouble!*"

I tried not to think about my own visual image. I mean, let's be realistic here: I'm bent over a massage table trussed and tied up with green cellophane like a Thanksgiving turkey.

Markus whispered in my ear, "Go inside, princess. Have a beautiful trip."

And then he started to run my Magic Wand vibrator all over my body. Markus used the plain, industrial-looking thing to visit the back of my neck and down the length of my body right to my feet. A feather danced from my ears to my toes. There was a sand-papery glove that he used to massage me again from stem to stern. He brushed and polished me. There was not a part of my body that didn't feel alive.

I was so aware of my every curve, I could not escape myself. Why is it that when I am blindfolded and stripped of my own movement, I find myself more connected to my own physical being than when I am "free"?

I was beginning to howl. Markus pushed something into my mouth. "Bite on this," he ordered. "Don't drop it."

I clamped my teeth into the balled-up rag and growled through it as Markus pumped up the music. I never felt safer in my life.

Thwack! Crack! I was being visited by the flogger. Markus was not playing.

He was insistent. The blows were coming fast and furious, pulling the breath from me. When I was about to shout "Yellow," the leather fingers of the flogger started to playfully bounce on my skin. I could feel Markus's body close to mine from behind. I could feel the leather chaps near my bottom. And then he started to massage my ass.

I could feel him holding big handfuls of my flesh. I felt warm oil dripping down my back as Markus began to move deeper.

I felt him lean over my body again. His heat was enough to send me over the edge. Then his mouth was right next to my ear as he whispered:

I love myself the way I am, there's nothing I need to change.
I'll always be the perfect me, there's nothing to rearrange.
I'm beautiful and capable of being the best me I can.
And I love myself just the way I am. I love you just the way you are.
There's nothing you need to do.
When I feel the love inside myself,
It's easy to love you.
Behind your fears, your rage and tears,
I see your shining star.
And I love you, just the way you are.

The tears ran down my cheeks. And Markus did something that I don't think he had ever done before. He placed little kisses on my neck and on my back and then began to tug and pull on the cellophane once more. He squeezed, spanked, and tickled. I was in a sweat and I couldn't keep that rag in my mouth one more second. I wanted to scream.

My mind had left the building and my body was taking me on a journey through the stars.

Time had stopped when the sound of scissors cutting away the cellophane brought me back to the here and now. Markus kept my blindfold on as he led me to a hot bath. He offered me water and asked me to just rest. "You have been on quite a trip, beautiful. Just take some time here and savor the journey."

I lay back in the warm water, and the image of myself naked on the cliff floated back to me. I had that same sense of wonder that I felt in New Mexico. She wasn't gone. I just had to reach for her.

Markus poked his nose into the bathroom and announced that we were having a luncheon celebration: homemade bento boxes. They must have taken him hours to prepare. They were almost too beautiful to eat.

"You know, I don't do this for all my clients." The Tiger grinned. "You're my special girl."

After a couple of sakes, full and wrapped in a warm robe, I was putty. That's when Markus dropped the bomb.

"I'm leaving for six weeks to take the Sexological Body Work certification course in SF," he said.

"The Sexological *what*? What is that and what the hell does it mean? Six weeks?" My dream state shattered. I realized just how dependent I'd become on him.

"I'm going to become a somatic sex educator. It's teaching people to integrate themselves through their bodies. It's what I've been doing with you all along, Pam," Markus said. "This work is powerful and I want to take it deeper. Joseph Kramer himself is leading the course."

I mulled it over. Even though I was scared of being without him, I understood. In fact, the thought of taking the training myself was intriguing. But that wasn't going to happen. At least not right now.

"Pammy, I'm going to be gone for quite a while. I want you to think about working with a friend of mine, Hank. He's got all your favorite qualities. He's gay. He's got great hands and is well respected in the community. He's even a licensed psychotherapist. Not many of those around in this work. He's great."

What else could I do except panic.

Chapter Twenty-Five
Women Loving Women

The house was a wreck. Everybody was home. Gavin was on the terrace stringing up the holiday lights. Andrew, back for winter break, and Ben were in their room, embroiled in one of their raging debates, which these days were about public policy instead of yesterday's Power Rangers versus Ninja Turtles. My mother was coming by for afternoon coffee. I thought my head would explode.

The walled-up compartments of my life were leaking. The intimacy I had with Markus felt overwhelming, especially now that I was going to have to manage without it for a month and a half. I needed to do something. Six weeks felt like forever. I caved. I was alone in the kitchen and called Hank. He was sensible, sophisticated, intellectually astute, and educated. There was not a hint of airy-fairy Daka-land in his voice. That was different. I liked it and set up an appointment for a couple of weeks later.

No sooner had I hung up when my mother burst in, took one look at the chaos, and began her inquisition. "What's going on? You're never around anymore. What are you up to? I'm not used to voice mail."

"Yeah, Mom, what are you up to?" Ben and Andrew said in unison, the Greek chorus emerging from their den.

"Whaddaya mean? It's always the same." I got defensive. "I'm under the gun with funding crunches, understaffing, the usual crises."

I could feel my mother coming in for the kill. She knew something was up, but I wasn't going to say one more word.

Andrew grabbed my arm and pulled me into his room.

"Hey, Mom, what's going on?" he whispered with urgency.

"What do you mean, kiddo?" I responded. I tried to keep things light. But I could feel the sweat beading my forehead. Had he broken into my secret e-mail account? Had that little scamp read my e-mails?

"Well, Mom, I don't know. Lately you've been different."

I crossed my arms and leaned, ever so nonchalantly, against the dresser.

"Different?" My voice cracked. "Different? How do you mean different? Different in a good way? Or different in a bad or strange way?"

"I dunno, you seem, well, happy! More independent in a lot of ways," Andrew said, and what had really been on his mind came out in a torrent. "There are all these weird books around the house! And those DVDs! You know, you could hide some of that stuff and not leave it around!"

Andrew's eyes practically rolled back in his head.

"You mean the educational sex DVDs like *Fire in the Valley*? Or *Extended Orgasm for Women*? Those DVDs?" (Subtext: "Isn't this the usual family-entertainment fare? Surely you're not talking about these old things?")

"Yes, Mom! *Those* DVDs!" (Subtext: "You're nuts.")

"Well, Andrew, you're sexually active and you have been for a long time. I just thought if I left those DVDs around you might actually watch them! If you're going to have sex, you might as well have great sex and learn how to be a better lover for your girlfriend and for yourself." I was on a Riverdale Goddess roll. Inappropriate? Perhaps. But honest.

"Your father and I don't want to separate sexuality from all the other things that we believe are essential for a fulfilled life. We keep all kinds of information for you and your brother. It's important."

"That's great, Mom, and I appreciate it." Andrew was actually sincere. "But I don't like them all over the kitchen table. I get embarrassed when I have someone over. Couldn't you create a special spot and I'll know where they are? A place not so out in the open? I just don't want my girlfriend accidentally picking up *Fire on the Mountain* or *Anal Massage Two.* You know what I mean?"

I took pity.

"Okay, Andrew. You know the drawer under the TV set in the living room? I'll keep all those DVDs there. That'll be our family's sex-info drawer."

Ben chose that moment to return from the bathroom. "Yeah, right. The sex drawer." The thought of it cracked up Ben, who had never said a word to me about the DVDs before. He turned to his brother. "Thanks for having the 'sex talk' with Mom. Saved me the grief." Then he looked at me. "Really, Mom. Justin was over the other day and he couldn't stop staring at the, ahem, 'cover art' of *Making Friends With Your G-Spot.* It was hard to concentrate on *World of Warcraft* with *that* in his face."

Andrew cut him off. "Don't sweat it, Mom. You're the best. I really do appreciate you offering us all of this stuff. You're way more open than a lot of other parents." Andrew was using the patient voice that I've used to explain things like there is no Santa Claus. My poor kids.

"Andrew, I get it. But you know those are all instructional DVDs, not porn, right?"

"Uh-huh. Right, Mom. Sure. No worries," Ben said, giving me a hug.

Andrew and I left Ben in the bedroom. He searched my face for reassurance before he said, "If you ever want to talk to me about what's going on in your life, Mom, I want you to know that you can!"

I wasn't aware that my inner revolution was perceptible to my kids. "Well, I am learning more about myself these days and I'm feeling better than I have in a long time. It's all good. You don't have to worry. Okay, honey?"

"Okay, Mom, okay. Just put the books and the DVDs in the special drawer. Like now, okay!" He scratched big quotation marks in the air when he said "special." I hated that. But he was so cute. Hopefully, he won't need too many years of therapy.

Mercifully, the phone rang. It was Corinna. She was turning out to be one of the most interesting women I knew, what with her Ivy League PhD and sexology certificate. "What's up with your friends?" she said. "I've been holding Body Erotic workshop spaces open for them. I need to know if they're coming next week."

"Beth and Sophia are coming. I'm sorry, I forgot to call to let you know."

"Great. So what are you doing tonight? I'm going to something you might find really interesting. Something you don't get to see every day. Are you game?"

"What is it?"

"It's a 'submit party,' an all-girl thing around themes of dominance and submission. Tonight, they're going to have a rope-tying demonstration."

Now, how could I turn that down? I felt so sophisticated and worldly. I was game to see what it was all about. No judgment from me, just healthy curiosity. The last female party I went to was all about the Tupperware.

I told Gavin my new friend Corinna had invited me out for the evening, some kind of all-girl event.

"And who is this Corinna person?" he asked.

I explained that she was a psychologist I met who was very involved with female sexuality. "In fact, she's conducting an all-women's sexuality workshop next weekend and I'm planning to go. So are Beth and Sophia. Corinna's so smart I thought maybe I could get her to write for the organization."

Already, I was telling him more than I ever had. Not quite the truth, but closer. My mother gave me the all-knowing eye. She scared the crap out of me sometimes.

I left the house, picking up Corinna on the way downtown. She identified as queer, which in her case translated to a hetero marriage and an attraction to women. She seemed to know about everything in the New York City Sacred Sexuality scene. She was unabashedly adventurous, edgy, and more than a little defiant. I found myself looking up to her, wanting her approval.

We arrived at a nondescript door on Houston Street. My first real sex club! There was nothing soul-searching in this adventure. I was merely a curious tourist. We checked in with a twentysomething with piercings in her eyebrow and nose, spiky hair, suspenders, and a tailored men's shirt. Corinna gave her the secret handshake. We read and signed a waiver and paid the fifteen bucks to get in the door.

Inside the club, a hostess ushered us into a sitting area. There was a coat check and a TV playing lesbian porn. A coffee table groaned with Twinkies, Ring Dings, chips, dips, and pretzels. A bunch of women were hanging out, chatting like it was an Alpha Delta Pi meeting and they were there to scope out the pledges.

There were so many kinds of women of every age, all decked out in latex or leather bondage gear, or corsets, or not much at all. What struck me most is that every possible body type was on display. Toned little bodies in French maid costumes, and one woman who easily weighed three hundred pounds in a tutu and striped leggings. Some had cue ball heads and some had flowing locks. In this space, there were no rules for feminine beauty.

Corinna and I were eager to get to where the action was, so we headed into the "play" area, discreetly hidden behind a black velvet curtain.

It was like an otherworldly stage set from a whacked-out production of *A Midsummer Night's Dream.* The ceiling was draped in branches that dripped leaves. Play spaces lined the wall, where people acted out their sexual fantasies—everything from a barred prison room to a doctor's office that spotlighted the examination table. If you had a fantasy, this was the perfect playground to explore it.

I found the women glorious! Did I mention that? I loved how accepting they were of each other.

There was a couple in the back of the club. One of the ladies was on all fours and wearing a dog collar while her lover pleasured her and spanked her from behind. Oh my! Her lover dominated her with such precision and patience. I found it so damn hot to watch these two women. And I was fascinated with myself for being a shameless voyeur and finding them so incredibly sexy. Where were those feelings coming from? Maybe Corinna was right. Perhaps sexual energy was simply sexual energy. Could it be that sexual energy was genderless?

And then there were two women who were bigger than big. I recognized Tutu Lady from the waiting room. She was now with her girlfriend, who was of equal girth and dressed in old-time military officer regalia. The Captain was on her knees, buried deep under the tutu, furiously pleasuring her girlfriend with her mouth. Tutu Lady was screaming in ecstasy. They were deeply engrossed in their sexual heat, oblivious to the gathering crowd. Maybe they got off on the attention. I was riveted.

Everywhere I looked, there were women touching each other, making public love. I didn't know that women had this kind of hot sexual aggression. It felt somehow masculine to me. I'd only seen men behave this way. I'd never ever seen women in the throes of raw sexual pleasure, so different from the faux ecstasy of porn flicks where women performed for men. This was real. These women loved each other. And I loved watching.

Partners were so patient and insistent about the pleasure they were giving to one another. No one was in a hurry to climax. They wanted to make their partners scream in extended orgasm. They loved the vulva! They celebrated the vulva! I was in awe. It made me appreciate fully for the first time how deeply sexual women could be. It made me want to celebrate being a woman.

Wow! I was wrong, this was no mere tourist excursion. It was one of the most mind-blowing experiences of my life. On the way out, I told Corinna: "I never knew there were so many different flavors of female sexuality. Do you think it's possible for women to be that uninhibited with men? I wanna be that free."

"You can be. It just takes patience and time. I know about this," she answered. "Trust me, you're on your way."

Chapter Twenty-Six

A New Hankering

As usual, I was stuck in rush-hour traffic on the West Side Highway at the end of the workday. My Altima was my mobile office and I'd just done four back-to-back interviews about the latest ethical eruption in the fertility field. A story had broken about a West Coast center that offered big bucks to "desirable" college women for their eggs. I had a lot to say about that, and none of it was pretty. My concentration was off, though. Half my mind was in Riverdale, worried that my Crock-Pot experiment might explode pulled pork all over the kitchen. The other half was filled with the image of the three-hundred-pound woman in her tutu with her "General." The three-ring circus that was my life was fatiguing yet magical. How did I do it all? Even now I was headed for new territory, with Hank. I found a little more room in my brain to begin to fantasize about what it might be like to meet this guy. I was lost in reverie when the cell phone beeped again. Shit. I needed a minute to myself. I screened the call, but how could I pass up Beth?

"Yo, babe," I said in greeting.

"Hey, goddess," Beth said in unison with Sophia, whom she

had conferenced in. Within seconds, they were pumping me for every second of the submit party.

"Let me just tell you this, these women's sexuality was incredible and bigger, lighter, noisier than I ever thought any sexuality could be. I felt like they'd given me permission to have desire and go for it. No apologies. No excuses. Not only did they fuck publicly, they ate in public. And I'm not talking carrot sticks. I'm talking Ring Dings. Those skinny bitches in the focus group would have had a stroke."

"Ring Dings? Really? Oh, my whole life I have loved those," Beth moaned.

"Uh-huh. And Twinkies, too."

"Why do you think I live with a woman?" Sophia said with a sexy, all-knowing laugh.

"It made me even more curious about Corinna's workshop this weekend," I said.

"Hell, I'm only willing to do this weekend because it is all women," Beth said. "Don't scare me."

"I just hope it doesn't snow. And, oh yeah, one more thing, just so you know: I'm testing the truth waters with Gavin. I told him about the workshop."

"That's a relief, since I'm going to be bunking at your place. One less thing I have to keep secret. It'll take the edge off for me," Beth said. "It's a good start for you, Pam."

"Thanks, guys, for coming with me. It means the world to me that you're willing to try out what's become an important part of my life. And how are you both doing?"

After a brief rundown—Beth's new exhibit at the gallery, Sophia starting to think about retiring—I said, "Sorry, girls, I gotta go."

"What's the big hurry, Pammy?" asked Sophia.

"I'm about to have a session with a new therapist Markus

recommended, and I'm late. It's been one helluva day. I was at the ABC-TV studio at five this morning and they actually forgot me in the greenroom! The phone's been ringing off the hook about the college-girl egg scandal. God, I hope this guy Hank is as good as Markus says he is. I need it. I'll call you later."

I parked and ran to Hank's midtown Manhattan building. I rang his buzzer and hoofed it up the four flights of stairs. I hate New York City walk-ups. I was sweating in my sheepskin Uggs by the time Hank greeted me at his door with a great big smile. He was a good-looking middle-aged man with a receding hairline, graying mustache, and toned body. He wasn't a jungle boy. No sarongs for him. Just functional sweatpants and a tank top. He exuded a sexy confidence and seductive intelligence. Yet he was grounded in reality and I felt in my bones that he was safe. I loved that his peephole cover on the door was a VAGINAS WELCOME button.

"C'mon in and we'll talk for a while. Get to know each other a little," Hank offered. I followed him into his book-lined living room, where we sat and chatted. Maybe because he was a psychotherapist he knew how to help me open right up about everything. Even about my work with Markus. It was different than telling my girlfriends. He was a part of the Sacred Intimacy world and he understood the depth of what I was achieving. I told him that I'd be taking the upcoming Body Electric workshop and how for the first time I was letting my husband in on what I was doing.

"I haven't told him all the details yet, but I'm planning to. I want to tell him everything. Actually, when I think about it, I want to tell the world. This work has such power to help people make peace with their pasts and make peace with themselves as they are. I never could have imagined feeling this whole before. It doesn't happen all the time, but there are moments when I feel like I'm touching God when I do this work. All this because I wanted a little erotic romp. Who knew? The thing is, I want everyone to have at least the chance to experience this. Sacred Intimacy needs to come aboveground."

"So you're a bit of a crusader," Hank said.

"I guess I am. I have a long history. I spoke out about infertility when it was so taboo everybody called it voodoo. Even today I was interviewed over and over again on a very touchy subject. I speak out. It's what I do. I have a reputation for saying the things that other people might think but don't have the guts or are too polite to say. Why shouldn't I do this with Sacred Sexuality? It's huge for me. I had no idea I was afraid of myself until I started this. I'm not so scared anymore."

Hank suppressed a laugh. "You have been on quite the journey, Pam. Not everyone would have the courage to face themselves this way. I guess if you're going to launch the next sexual revolution, you better tell your husband."

"It's on the agenda, Hank. But I want more."

"So let me see if I've got this right. You would really feel seen if you were able to share this part of yourself with the world, wouldn't you?"

The minute he said that, I realized it was true. I wanted the new, integrated, sexual me to come out and be embraced. I knew I risked rejection, but I wasn't going to let it stop me. Every time I got naked, physically or emotionally, I felt vulnerable and scared. Nothing terrified me more than being judged. But over the past six months, I had learned that it was never as bad as I thought it was going to be, and I thrived. It was part of my healing.

Hank picked up on the vibe. "Why don't we make today's session about being seen?"

I had a moment of hesitation. Up they came again, all the old issues about my weight and body. Instead of holding on to embarrassment, I noticed it, gave myself a reassuring mental hug, and let it go. I got undressed and climbed up on the table, facedown. It was amazing that after all my experience, this first step was still so hard. I did what I always do—I focused on the music and breathed.

Hank got me out of my head and into my body in record time. I relaxed into my familiar place on the table and got lost in the pleasure of his hands. I started to feel free. I began to move in time to the pulsing rhythms that filled the room, and he urged me on. "That's right. Feel it all. That's right. You're doing great."

I let myself play with my hair and touch my body. The goddess was back. She'd bumped out the frightened fat girl. The only thing I felt in that moment was wildly beautiful. I forced open my eyes a slit because I wanted to witness myself being seen just like this. Hank's eyes were waiting. If they were hands, they would have caught me.

"Come on, open them wider. Look at me," Hank encouraged. I did, and I saw all I wanted: loving acceptance.

Emboldened, I did something I'd never done before. I got up onto my knees and danced, swaying and rocking to the beat. I reached for him. Hank wrapped his arms around me, holding me, supporting me, and finally joining me in my table dance. We were uninhibited, playful, and happy. We danced so close that I was in his lap, face-to-face, his hands clasping my waist.

Old habits die hard. The worry that I'd once again gone too far, that I was too big, clutched my heart.

"Am I too much for you?" I asked, holding my breath.

He pulled me to him until there was no space between us. "Honey, does it feel like I can't hold all of you?" Hank breathed into my ear, tightening his grip. "I am a big boy. I can take care of myself—your job here is not to worry about any of that. I have you."

The breath left my lungs in a shuddering sigh and I let him cradle me until . . . there I was, back in traffic heading home to my Crock-Pot. Now, that's what I call a day's work.

Chapter Twenty-Seven

Celebrating the Body Erotic

I WAS GATHERING MY stuff together for the women's workshop, stepping over shopping bags filled with our interfaith blend of holiday presents. Beth was running a few minutes late. Gavin watched me race around packing up pillows, towels, and snacks that were on the suggested list. When I asked him where Ben's sleeping bag was, he finally said something.

"What the hell are you doing? Are you girls camping out tonight? You told me this was in an office building downtown."

"It is. There's apparently a lot that we need in order to be comfy. Celebrating the Body Erotic is going to be hard work," I said, deciding against the sleeping bag and opting for the Back Jack instead.

"Yeah, right. A bunch of women talking about their feelings, you do that all the time. You've been training for this your whole life. Me? I'd rather have my chest waxed."

"What do you know? Did you even check out the link I sent you for the workshop? They have them for men, too." I was warming him up for the big reveal.

He burst out laughing. "I read it, Pam. Honestly, this is not for me. But you girls, go knock yourselves out. Have fun," he said, handing me a great big duffel bag to carry it all. He patted my head and pecked my cheek as I left the house.

Even with the late start, we got to the workshop an hour early. Sophia was hungry, so we searched the Wall Street neighborhood for a coffee shop. The financial district, bursting with life during the workday, was emptying out for the weekend. The streets were taking on a Dickensian look as the beautiful but dirty building facades shut down and the lights in the windows went dark. Our usual martinis called to us, but we had sworn to remain alcohol-free the whole weekend. We took refuge in the only nonbar that was open on a Friday evening, Starbucks, and sipped eggnog lattes while we nibbled on scones. Not quite the rush we were looking for, but better than nothing.

"I read the workshop description and I'm fine with it. But I'm not gonna work on either of you. I'd rather 'practice giving sensual touch' on someone I don't ever have to see again." Beth was joking but she wasn't kidding.

"No worries," I said. "I arranged with Corinna and Max, the leader, to put us in different groups when there's hands-on work. It'll be fine."

"I'm so relieved." Beth exhaled. "And excited. I'm doing something new. I need to shake off my life for a couple of days. Everything has been feeling stale. This, on the other hand, feels a little bit edgy. I like it."

"And sexy," Sophia added. "Don't forget sexy."

"I'm glad you're excited," I said. "I know I'm the instigator, but this is really new for me, too, and I'm happy you're both here. I've never worked with women before."

"Just keep an open mind." Sophia grinned.

We finished up and headed to the workshop. Just as we walked into the office suite where guys in custom-made suits ordinarily turned multi-billion-dollar deals, I made the decision to tell them.

"You know, girls, I'm thinking I have to write about all this."

Before they could pick their jaws off the ground, Max, a surprisingly handsome woman full of male energy, called the workshop to order. She asked us to sit on the floor in the inevitable circle. As we had agreed, Beth, Sophia, and I split up so that we wouldn't get in each other's way. We all wanted our own experience. I sat down between a heavyset African queen with a shaved head and long, dangly earrings and a Wal-Mart grandma whose hip required a chair. About thirty of us gathered. We were a gorgeous mosaic of white, black, yellow, and brown; some of us in our early twenties and others as old as seventy. We were thin. We were fat. We were a mix of blue- and white-collar workers. In the end, we were simply a group of women coming together to explore something uniquely female.

While everyone got settled, I took in the space. Corinna was bustling about, managing the volunteers from the Body Electric, the organization that ran the Celebrating the Body Erotic program. Under her iron fist, they'd turned the testosterone banker space into a beautiful, almost haremlike setting with sarongs hanging from the walls and flowers everywhere. There was a table of snacks and drinks. Massage tables were stacked in a corner next to boxes of surgical gloves, oils, and lube. That made me wonder just how intimate we girls were going to get. Beth and Sophia took it all in, too, and were looking a bit green around the gills.

It hit me then what a brave and determined lot we were. It took a lot of nerve for each one of us to show up at an empty office building at seven on a Friday night to explore ourselves. And we all plunged in with an openness that took my breath away.

Max had us gather around her as she talked about all the words that society uses to describe our genitals and asked us to pitch in with names.

"Vagina," yelled out someone with an affinity for the obvious.

"Vulva," chimed in a would-be nurse.

"Va-jay-jay," giggled an Oprah fan.

"Oh yeah, and then there's my fave, twat," another one growled.

"Cunt," snarled a tough-looking woman.

Max stopped us right there.

"I like to use the word 'cunt' because it's a word that has been taken from us women," she said. "It's been turned into a negative, an expletive, when in fact 'cunt' means 'holy well.'"

She sat back and looked at us expectantly, gauging our reactions. Then Max said, "Dearies, today each of you is going to start using the term that works for you. Just to make sure we all know what we're talking about, we're going to the land down under for a geography lesson."

The room quaked with curiosity. While she had us riveted, Max immediately dropped her pants and told us she was going to model for us.

Max was something to behold. She had tribal tattoos running across her pelvis; they were bold, dark, and ancient-looking. Her pubic hair was untamed and untrimmed. Me? I hardly had any pubic hair left, styling myself in the manner of the genital fashionistas. All I had left was a neat little patch of dark hair.

Max was sitting on the floor with her legs spread and the class gathered around. She held a hand mirror to reflect herself so she could guide us accurately.

"Vulvas, yonis, cunts, whatever you call them, are all like flowers," Max said gently as she explored her own nether region and shared her most private feelings about this powerful body part. "No two are alike. Some women have big inner labia; others have labia so small they're almost nonexistent. The clitoris, too, ranges in size. They are all normal and wonderful."

It was profound and surprisingly moving. When she had completed the intimate tour, she announced that we were going to have our own chance to show and tell. There was a deafening shuffle. Discomfort and embarrassment took hold. But not for long.

Max and Corinna set up a "throne," a Back Jack with a towel draped over it. Max called for volunteers. The room went quiet. Until I piped up.

"Okay," I said, "I'll do it. I'll go first." What else is new?

I put my towel on the "throne" and Corinna supported my back as I opened my legs and revealed my yoni. That's the name I chose for my vulva that day. The Sanskrit translation sounded so soft.

I glanced up into a field of amazed, curious, and admiring eyes. I sucked in some air and held up the mirror to the face of my femaleness. The words just came.

"I used to think that vulvas were ugly, wrinkled things that were not meant to be looked at. And I was sure that mine was probably the ugliest of all. But I'm surprised. I don't feel that anymore. I actually like that I can see so much of my yoni now with my pubic hair mostly gone."

That's how I began to talk about this anatomical part that was so secret and fetishized that I never even thought to talk about it at all, except with my gynecologist. And even then it was under a sheet.

"Pubic hair was always a thing for me. How much to have. Trimming it back felt like hacking back a forest. And at the gym, I noticed how all the younger women had their pubic hair lasered, waxed, or shaved to the point of being bald or almost bald. Having this big hairy bush made me feel old and obsolete."

I was absently petting what was left of my pubic hair while I talked.

"I wanted a more updated model. So I went and had myself lasered. Allegedly permanent, definitely painful and expensive. But after I did it, I could actually see my yoni for the first time. It just about knocked me off my feet. I could see my inner labia. It was like, 'Hello, labia! How are you? Look at you! You are out there, aren't you?' I now understood why some women put rings in them. In my opinion, the inner labia need dressing up, especially without pubic hair to give them cover! You can see that my inner labia are kind of big."

I heard some giggles and glimpsed nods of understanding from some of the women. Encouraged, I looked deeper inside of me and exposed my clit. It was such an odd mix of vulnerability and safety among these women.

"My clit has always made me happy. I don't like it when some 'sexperts' say that clitoral orgasms are 'less mature' than G-spot orgasms. I feel that my clit has always been mature and worthy."

Then I looked deeper at my vaginal opening. Sadness hit me like a lightning bolt.

"I remember a time when I felt that my vagina had let me down during my struggle with infertility. The experience disconnected me from my whole reproductive and sexual self. I felt that my vagina had betrayed me by not offering to readily conceive. That was a hard time. When I finally got pregnant, my vagina betrayed me again. It wouldn't open enough to let my sons pass through. My belly needed to be cut because Miss Vagina wouldn't cooperate. It was so painful. I was so angry at my own body. But time has gone by, and my vulva and I have long ago made up. Still, that memory is raw."

At this point, I was weepy and talking more to myself than to the assembled group. I had a lot to say. I mean, it isn't like we get much opportunity to chat about our genitals.

"I like that part of me. I can feel it better in its naked state. I love that so much more of me is open to touch without the hair. I love that I have made peace with my funny big labia and my big clit. I guess I should say thank you for all the pleasure and for helping to give me my boys."

With that I gave up the mirror, grabbed two tissues, and smiled at my sympathetic audience. I relinquished the throne to the next plucky female, as another woman touched my arm and whispered, "I was so relieved to see you. All these years I thought I was deformed and really I look just like you."

I burst into tears all over again. I hugged her. "I know. It's so hard being all alone with your body with nothing real to compare it to. How can we ever match the Photoshopped images we see in *Playboy*? Why the hell should we, anyway?"

It was a charged and emotional night. When we got back to the car, I was still lost in the drama of the show-and-tell when Beth exploded.

"Are you out of your mind? Writing about this? Is that what you said before? Have you thought about all those straitlaced fertility docs you work with? Can't you just hear the hot gossip at their next annual conference?"

Sophia jumped right in. "Yeah, Pam. Imagine them standing in line patiently waiting for their free lattes, pens, and stress balls from big pharma, yukking it up. 'Hey, did you read page seventy-five where Pamela has raspberries in her p-p-pu-u-ssy?'"

Cackling, Beth deepened her voice. "'Nope, didn't get to that part yet. I'm still trying to picture Pamela with her panties down, bent over that guy's knee, getting her ass whacked! I know people who would pay good money to do that to her.'"

"'Talk about a fund-raiser! Ha ha ha!'" Sophia quipped.

I felt my color rising. Maybe they were right. I didn't think I could stand them making fun of me. I wasn't sure I could risk the humiliation. I knew I wasn't that strong. Yet.

"Okay, I got it. Point taken. I need to think more about this." I grew quiet as they chattered about the experience of that night. My heart rate was just getting back to normal when Beth circled back.

"Listen, my budding author, I don't mean to tease you to death, but slow down. Don't you think you need to tell Gavin before you tell the world?"

"Yes, I do, Beth. And tonight's the night."

"When I'm there? There's no place to hide at your place. If you need me, I'll be taking a three-hour shower."

Beth and I swept into the apartment, the very embodiment of goddess energy.

Gavin was working on his laptop and greeted us with open curiosity. "So, how did the workshop go? What did you do?" He wanted to know. This was good, I thought. At the same time, I wasn't sure how to explain my evening in a way that wouldn't sound just plain weird. Max had warned us to be careful about telling anyone, even our intimate partners and friends, about the experience. "If you're not in the room, it can be awfully hard to understand."

After about five minutes of my enthusiastic monologue, Gavin's face twisted in disgust. "You mean you got naked with all of these women? Did they touch you? You showed them your vagina? Were they all lesbians?"

I thought he was going to infarct.

"Not all lesbians. Just some." I was sinking into defensiveness. "Yes, I showed them my vagina and it was one of the most therapeutic things I've ever done."

Max was right. This was a bad idea.

He cut me off. He was visibly twitching. "I can't believe it. How could you let women touch you and look up your vagina?"

Gavin being upset threw me. It was all women, for God's

sakes. He was on a rant. "What's left? What are you going to do tomorrow, give each other happy endings?"

I was so taken aback I lost any words and the tears welled up. If I couldn't tell him about this, how could I tell him about everything else I'd been up to? My bravado dissolved.

At that moment, Beth burst out of the bathroom, glowing. Gavin turned on her.

"So I understand your friendship with Pam reached a whole new level today. How was that for you? Did your vagina have a story to tell, too?"

"Oh shut up, G. What do you know?" Beth snapped, hurling a pillow at his head.

Chapter Twenty-Eight

My Big Fat Lesbian Experience

I WOKE UP AFTER a nearly sleepless night, nervous about coming out to Gavin. I knew there was no choice. It was a matter of timing. But at least I could spare Beth the scene. I nudged her into consciousness with a cup of scalding black coffee, careful not to wake the sleeping dragon or the boys, and dragged her out for Day Two.

It began like all other workshops: in a freaking circle. We processed. We cried. We talked about how misunderstood we were. Two women didn't come back. We had to process that, too. It seemed we'd all told someone about the previous day's activities to no good effect. Max tried to keep the outpouring under control. Two hours later, we got down to business.

We spent several hours in teams of three working on the practical skills required for the art of sensual, not erotic, massage. We studiously avoided genitals and only minimally, if ever, touched breasts. I took to giving massage like a fish to water. I'd had so many rich private sessions that I had a good idea of what it should look and feel like. Giving someone a fantastic experience on the table made me feel powerful.

Touching another woman's naked body in a remotely sensual way, though, tested my limits. As savvy as I'd become, it still made me anxious. But after five minutes of working on a beautiful, abundant thirtysomething Latina with a great ass, I completely forgot about anything other than the body at hand. I was rocked by the fact that I was feeling more than a little turned on by the pleasure I was giving to her.

It was all good prep for the grand finale: full-blown erotic massage. Gavin was going to love this one.

Max said, "Don't be surprised if you have an emotional release of some kind. Many people go into deep erotic trances during these massages. Some need to cry, laugh, or scream. And some people go on colorful trips in their bodies as they float around the universe for a while, having visions or hearing messages."

Tell me something I didn't know.

"Do you get the munchies afterward?" I piped up. Such a class cutup.

Max shot me a look and asked one of the Body Electric volunteers to get undressed and climb onto a massage table for the demo. Beth, Sophia, and I traded looks across the room and simultaneously mouthed a big "wow."

"Dearies, hygiene comes first," said Max, snapping on a pair of latex gloves. She was an old hand at this.

She talked gently to the heroic volunteer, showing us how to make someone feel secure when they're naked and exposed. She demonstrated the soft touch to use at the beginning. Max showed us all the different ways to touch a breast to give a woman pleasure.

"As for the vulva, we should approach it only when we're welcomed there." Max was a flawless multitasker. Somehow she managed to convey all this information while she kept the volunteer in a state of intimate warmth. It was amazing to watch Max's hands as she demonstrated the many different strokes that the vulva liked.

"Some women love inner labia shiatsu massage," Max instructed. "And some women like soft drumming, like this. And remember, dearies, lube is good."

I was trying to get a closer look. I wasn't the only one. All of us were straining to see better, as if we'd never seen a vagina before. We were all captivated. The Discovery Channel had nothing on this. I knew Beth, Sophia, and I would be talking about this forever.

Max and Corinna again divided us into groups of threes. I was a receiver to start and I got to choose the two women who would work with me. Gotta admit, despite the tutorial, I was still nervous about the girl-on-girl thing. It felt way safer for me to give than to get. But I made up my mind that I'd just relax and go with the flow. I kept reminding myself about the glories of the submit party and how turned on I had felt watching those ecstatic women.

What the hell. I got up on the table and was immediately distracted by the activity around the room. I couldn't focus on my body, so I asked for one of the bandannas that were offered as blindfolds. Seems I wasn't the only one who needed help concentrating. Once I blocked out the visions, I had no trouble traveling inside myself.

My teammates' hands may not have been professional, but they were sweet and loving. They asked permission to touch, inquiring how I was feeling all along the way. And I kept thinking, *So, this is how girl hands feel. They're softer and smaller.*

It wasn't all about muscle. These hands moved intuitively, as if they could anticipate what my body craved. These women were also in their own exploration, finding the joy of giving. We were journeying together into something brand-new.

Max's voice rang out. "It's time for us to think about closing and having the last bits of delicious touch."

Before I knew it, she was banging a drum, ending the session.

I found myself emerging from an altered state. I was floating on a cloud of rainbows. And I felt like I was hearing a voice inside my head telling me to love myself just as I am. That I was enough just as I was, and that there was nothing to achieve. No place that I had to go. (Markus? Is that you?)

My kaleidoscopic daydream fractured abruptly when I heard the weeping and howling that filled the space. So many of us were experiencing different kinds of profound emotion. It freaked me out. I was all opened up in my rainbow love-fest and it sounded like Armageddon was erupting around me. I curled up and tried to block it out. I got a real hit of the pain so many of us carry. I closed my eyes and said a prayer for us all.

The three of us left, exhausted and lost in thought. The car was quiet. I was deep in conversation with myself. In less than a year, I had gone from zero sexual exploration to showing my vulva to a group of women I'd just met. How did I get there?

Beth interrupted the silence. "Okay, I get this. It's all the things you say. It's profound. I looked at places in myself I had forgotten about. It was great being with the 'tribe,' but honey, I want the Tiger. And I want you to book it for me for my birthday."

"Alrighty then," said Sophia. "Speaking your desires, huh? You really did get with the program this weekend."

"Yeah and it's gonna cost me," I said. "E-mail me your schedule and I'll set it up first thing tomorrow. As for me, I'm going on a body-soul cleanse. Seriously cleaning out the old shit. No more white food and no more white lies. I'm telling Gavin. And you, Sophia, what's your big breakthrough?"

"Me? I'm sleeping in."

Chapter Twenty-Nine

One Last Bridge

I MADE GOOD ON my vow to clean myself up. Okay, it wasn't the next day, but it was January 1. How traditional. I was tearing through the cupboards with a big plastic garbage bag, throwing out all the things that I always relied on. White foods—crackers, pretzels (my personal crack cocaine), cookies, white rice—were all part of my cover-up. They were my emotional Band-Aids, what I reached for whenever I was feeling lonely, sad, angry, or even happy. Whenever I gave up comfort food before, it was to go on a diet. I was done with diets. After seven months of surrendering to my own truths, my Band-Aids had stopped working. I didn't need or want those empty calories, although it scared me a little—or maybe a lot—to see them go.

Fear wasn't going to stop me anymore. Just like I wouldn't let fear of Gavin's reaction stop me from telling him the truth. I'd do it when he got home from visiting his parents for their traditional New Year's Day brunch. I had begged off. I needed a reprieve from the Madsen clan after the Christmas marathon. I needed the time to pull up all the courage I had. The irony was that this particular surrender was exactly the kind of provocation that would normally send me headfirst into a bag of pretzels. Now that was no longer a possibility. I'd come too far. In my gut, I felt no shame. I wasn't blind—I knew that Sacred Intimacy, one-way touch, Tantra, and spanking opened me to all sorts of comments and criticisms. The thing is, I knew this work allowed me to become way more interesting, joyful, confident, and sexy than I had ever dared imagine I could be.

It was time to let Gavin in on what was happening to the woman he had married.

I was so busy rehearsing what I was going to say, I didn't notice Gavin standing in the kitchen doorway, grinning as he watched me toss out the unopened boxes of saltines, Chips Ahoy!, and Frosted Flakes.

"New diet?" Gavin grabbed my ass as I knelt in the pantry, searching for starch. I was so startled that I banged my head standing up before I let myself fall back into his arms. It felt so good. Did I want to rock our world, the world that he thought he knew so well?

"I don't smell anything cooking. We ordering in?" he asked.

I gathered my courage and turned to face him.

"Honey, I have something to tell you. And I want you to know that I love you."

"Pammy, are you sick? Honey?"

"No, Gavin. Nothing like that at all. It's just that I had been sinking, feeling stuck in my life. Stuck in my body. Stuck in my sexuality. Do you realize that you are the only man who's ever touched me in a sexual way? I just couldn't imagine that for my entire life."

I tried to look into Gavin's eyes, but he turned away. His face drained of color. I plowed on. "I didn't want to cheat on you. I love you. I didn't want to have an affair and fall in love with another man. I didn't want to tear our family apart. But I needed to feel touch and adventure in my life."

The speeches I'd practiced all afternoon were gone. I didn't know what was going to come out next. I just kept going.

"I want you to understand, this isn't about you at all," I said.

"Great. Isn't that how every breakup starts?" Gavin's face was white.

"Honey, this is not a breakup speech. I'm not leaving you and I hope you want me to stay. I want to tell you some things about me. About everything that's been changing for me."

"Okay . . . should I be sitting down?" His confusion made me ache. This wasn't going the way I wanted.

"You see, Gavin, I started out wanting only a safe sexual adventure. Nothing with nothing. But then it turned into something, a kind of healing for me. I started to work with several men—"

He cut me off. "Really! Men! Wow, that's a relief. Here I was worried that you were into women. After you spent a weekend muff-diving, how was I supposed to know you 'work' with men?"

I absorbed the burn of Gavin's sarcasm and waited while a succession of dark storms blew across his brow. I put my arm through his unyielding one and pulled him to the sofa. He wouldn't look at me, but he didn't pull away, either.

There was nothing to do but keep going. "These are experts, Gavin. Mostly gay men who work with sexual energy and sexual touch. It's called Sacred Sexuality. I can give you their Web sites and articles to read. I've learned so much and I want to share it all with you. It would be incredible for our marriage."

Before he could say anything else. I unloaded it all—the workshops, how these people helped me see my body differently and helped me with my food demons. I told him how, for the first time in a long time, I felt truly alive.

"I love you, Gavin. I need you to listen to me."

I watched his fingers twitch. They always twitched when his upset was bone deep. I wanted him to get it, to nod in understanding and wrap me in his arms. Pure fantasy. This was big. I had just lobbed grenades into his reality. I prayed Gavin could see they were unarmed. That we were intact. He stood up and walked back into the kitchen. I followed him and watched quietly while he banged together a sandwich, which he then abandoned on the counter. I dogged him back to the sofa, sitting so close to him that not a hair could come between us.

"Gavin, you are the only person that I have ever made love with." I was hoarse with fear and affection. "I'm not fucking anyone other than you. I'm not in love with anyone other than you. I am working with trained professionals. I pay for these services. That's all."

There was an excruciating pause. We sat side by side in silence until finally he said, "Just tell me that I'm not going to lose you."

"I don't want to lose you either," I murmured into his shirt. And he did what I longed for— he held me.

Gavin stroked my hair and kissed my eyes. "You are such a nut. I guess it's one of the reasons I love you," he said. "I'm not saying it's always easy. But it's never dull."

"Haven't you noticed how much I've changed lately? Don't you see how much happier I've been?" I knew I was pushing my luck, but I desperately wanted him to see. To see me.

"Well"—Gavin started to laugh—"you're not picking on me as much. That's good. You hardly ever get angry anymore. That's good, too. When I come to think about it, you've been pretty great. And you're not hitting the chips, either. Actually, you're looking beautiful. Yeah, I guess I've noticed. And all this time I thought it was new lipstick."

"C'mon back in the kitchen. I'll pour you a glass of wine and heat up the chili I made. I know you love my chili." I wanted to keep him close by me and continue the conversation. It was a relief to finally get my secret out. He hadn't threatened to take the children away or ship me off to a psychiatric institution. A good start. I was beginning to feel that maybe we could move forward together. I had no illusion that it wouldn't take some work. This didn't come naturally to Gavin; he wasn't a "process" kind of man. He was more a nail-and-hammer guy: If it's broke, fix it and don't whine. He was such a WASP, and a Nordic one at that. How he fell in love with a Jewish princess who talked all emotion all the time was one of life's great mysteries.

"I'd rather have a beer, hon," he said, coming up behind me. I bent into the fridge to get him a brew and he grabbed my butt and kissed my neck. It was a deliciously familiar affection that I was grateful for. We marinated in it for a while, letting the love push the upset into a corner.

I gazed into his smiling hazel eyes, and, never content to let a good thing be, said, "You know, sweetie, you'd look so hot with a shaved head and a goatee. Oooh, and an earring. So pirate."

He jerked back. "And you, Pamela, would look really hot with hair down to your ass. If you do that, maybe I'll shave my head."

Humph, I thought. For years, I wore my hair very long for him. Gavin loved long hair. I still wore it past my shoulders just to please him. But it would never be long enough for him. A big turn-on for Gavin was simply brushing my hair. Some men like big tits; Gavin liked big hair. Everybody's got their thing. Hell, I'd just learned that he really liked asses and I liked getting spanked.

No sooner had the thought entered my head than it was out of my mouth.

"Gavin, the man I mostly work with, his name is Markus. Well, Markus gave me a spanking in one of our last sessions."

Goddamn it, I see a pot and I just have to stir it. I didn't plan to talk about the details of my sessions. Ever. But I thought—if I could claim to be thinking at all—that if I opened up a bit more, we might get somewhere.

Gavin stopped with a mouthful of beer. I heard him swallow. "Really? And did you like that?"

"Yes, I liked it very much," I blurted out, and kept on going. "Actually, it was one of my best sessions."

He went for the chili bubbling on the stove and didn't look at me when he asked, "Pants up or down?"

I stopped breathing. "Actually, I was completely naked, honey. Not only was it really sexy, the experience opened me up in a way that I could never have imagined. The position I was in left me nowhere to hide. Everything about me was in the open. Just like right now. In that one session, I learned that if I can get over my shame about my own sexual desires, my fantasies, and express them, that there's the possibility of tremendous pleasure. More than that, when I got out of my own way, I began to come to terms with who I really am as a woman."

I paused and looked Gavin square in the eye. "Do you have a fantasy that you would like to experience?"

He was squirming and wolfing down the really spicy chili. He swallowed and spoke. "I don't know if acting out my fantasies is a good thing. I mean, maybe they are better left in my head and in movies. I think that I would be too embarrassed to share my fantasies. And what if I didn't like them in real life?"

There was a pregnant pause before he went on. "I think I'm okay with you doing this for yourself, baby, but I'm not sure this is for me."

Even though he wasn't running out the door, I could feel it closing. So I continued to push. "If you shared your desires with me, perhaps I could fulfill them for you. Or we could do a session with a trained sexologist together. How would that be?"

Gavin didn't answer my question directly, "Did you want Markus to spank you or did you just want to be spanked?"

Okay, that was a fair and yet complicated question. Was he feeling jealousy? Was this a trick question, and what if I got it wrong?

"I wanted both, Gavin. That's the truth. My sexual hot points have always included some kind of mild domination. I can say that now. Look at me! I've spent my life running the show! It is so sexy for me to not be in control. And I have always thought that spanking was incredibly sexy, especially certain kinds of spanking. But it was too shameful a request, so I buried it. It went against every hard-won feminist understanding I had. I couldn't tell you. I could barely admit it to myself. So yes, I really wanted an over-the-knee sustained spanking. And yes, in that moment, I really wanted Markus to be the one to give it to me. It felt safe. He knows what he's doing. And after all my sessions, I trust him completely."

"And just how many sessions have you had? How long has this been going on?"

I tried to gauge the way the wind was blowing. I put my wifely finger in the air. I sensed calm seas, not an angry tempest. "Quite a few. Many months."

Wow. I said the entire truth. Talk about living in transparency! Markus would be proud. The girls would be amazed.

"Did he spank you for a long time? What did he use?"

Now he was pushing my buttons. He wanted intimate details. This was harder than I thought. I felt color coming into my cheeks.

"Markus spanked me for a long time with his hand. We changed spanking positions a couple of times. Sometimes he took a break from the spanking and massaged me. He gave me some sensual and erotic touch, too. But the spanking was always a part of it. And he didn't always spank my bottom. Sometimes he spanked my legs and my back. I think to vary the sensation and to give my bottom a break."

"Okay, I got it," Gavin said. "Look, I don't know if I could do what you're doing. I don't know if I want to. And right now, I couldn't even tell you what my fantasies are. Maybe I could e-mail you some of the erotica I've kept to myself. You could read it and know what turns me on that way?" Gavin was stretching. My heart went out to him.

"That would be great, Gavin."

As difficult as all that was for me, I could see Gavin struggling with this whole new chapter of having me as a wife. I had turned from the regular Sunday chicken dinner to a "Wednesday's Surprise Special" pretty darn fast! Meanwhile, we were polishing off the chili.

I scraped the bottom of the pot with my finger, licking off the last bits. We piled the dirty plates, everything back to normal. Or so I thought.

"You know, Pam, I could spank you."

My first response was pure fear. The idea of an untrained spanker, especially one who might be carrying a little bit of resentment toward the spankee, made me queasy.

"Oh, that's so brave of you," I answered. "I know it's not your thing, though. Maybe we could find something else."

"No, no, no. I really want to do this for you." Gavin was insistent. "If this turns you on, I could at the very least give it a whack."

He thought he was so clever.

"Fine. But you need a few lessons first. There's an art to making this sexy. There are rules to the game. How about we do a session with Markus?"

What the hell is wrong with me? Did I really want Gavin in Markus's living room? I had to think about this. I wasn't at all sure

I wanted my men to meet. I had it all compartmentalized and neat. This could get messy. But the train was way out of the station.

"Sure, book it with Markus. How about this weekend?"

So I did. One for us and one for Beth. For Markus, it was Christmas—he was finally getting to meet the "Mister."

Chapter Thirty

Purple Passion

I SPENT A SLEEPLESS night, high on honesty. Transparency was rapidly becoming my drug of choice. It left me in a New Agey, feel-good cloud. After all the months of nagging, the gang deserved to know I'd come out. As soon as the apartment emptied in the morning, I called each one. There were whoops all around. There wasn't one who didn't want to marry Gavin.

"I guess you won't be needing that divorce attorney I found for you. Too bad. I hear he's gorgeous." Beth was always so supportive.

"Do you know how courageous Gavin is?" Olivia was awed. "My husband would be curled up in the fetal position."

"Gavin is pretty spectacular, isn't he?" I agreed. "And wrap your mind around this: He wants to do a session with me and Markus."

"You do understand that his willingness to do that is a testament to his love? People have killed for less. I adore him. I'm so glad you have him in your life." Cousin Sophia sighed, a die-hard Gavin fan from way back.

"So when are you going to tell Mom?" Vicki asked.

"After our session with the Tiger," I answered. "One beast at a time."

"Well, I want to be around when you do."

"Not a chance, Vic," I said. "But I'm sure you'll hear all about it. Instant replay."

Then I called Bitsy. She'd been so worried about the potential for radioactive fallout from my extramarital activities, it was only fair to let her know that Gavin and I survived the truth bomb.

"Gawd, Pam. That's a load off. I can't take another week of keeping this in the dark. I swear, the next time Gavin picked up the phone, I would've come out and told him myself. You know, I've been thinking a lot about one-way touch ever since you mentioned it. Maybe it is the way for me to resurrect my dead libido. The testosterone patches did nothing except get me into a fight with my plumber. The Tiger brought your sex drive back from the grave. I called him."

"You did? No, you didn't! Bits, that's fantastic."

"Will you meet me after my massage? I need to know you'll be waiting," she pleaded.

I promised, hung up, and got dressed to meet Bob, who had flown into town to strategize with me and the board about fund-raising for the next fiscal year. I hoofed it to the car for the stop-and-go traffic into Manhattan. It was the first chance I had to think seriously about how liberating and normalizing it was for me to be able to talk honestly with Gavin and all the people in my life. The thing I didn't anticipate was their eagerness to try it out. I was starting to feel like the Pied Piper of Sacred Intimacy. Hearing the echoes of Bitsy's excited voice, it dawned on me what a big responsibility it was. The last thing I needed was to take the blame for an on-table disaster. My friends were enticed by their fantasy of the Tiger experience. But I knew that this work could put you eyeball-to-eyeball with your demons. I was worried that they weren't prepared. I told myself to let go, they're all adults.

I made it to Chelsea in record time. I was on the dot. Bob was early, as usual. I found him sitting at the quietest table in our favorite bistro. His computer was propped open and there were piles of spreadsheets.

"Hey, Pam," he twanged. "I think I've got the next year figured out."

Over the next two hours, he attempted to deconstruct the numbers—not my strong point. I was big picture and he was detail, which made us a great team. When he was convinced that I was on solid enough ground to present the annual budget to the board, we took the break we'd been waiting for.

He went right for his "low carb" scotch on the rocks. I had my signature dirty martini. We both ordered salad and then dived into the good stuff. Poor Bob. He was starving in Texas. I spoon-fed him my latest sexplorations. He was salivating. I gave him more.

"I did it. I told Gavin. We're doing a session together," I went on breathlessly. "And guess what . . . you didn't hear this from me, but Bitsy and Beth are having a session, too."

"Together? Me likey."

I kicked him.

"Seriously, I wish I had the guts to do what you're doing with Gavin. I need to jump-start my relationship with Michael."

"Why don't you? You'll have the perfect opportunity when we go to San Francisco in February."

"And why is that?" Bob asked.

"Well, because you're going to be there anyway for a whole week. The environment and fertility conference is on Thursday and Friday. My speech is fabulous, by the way. Practice visits start on Monday. We get the whole weekend! I got upgraded to a suite at the

Queen Anne, so Beth is staying in my room. Markus is coming, too. He's going to see about becoming a certified teacher at the next Sexological Body Work class. I'm sure if you bring Michael in for a session, Markus will be happy to see you both. You can use my room. Beth and I won't mind clearing out."

Bob didn't miss a beat. He whipped out his phone and cleared the date with Michael right then and there.

He glowed with anticipation and I cheerfully counted off all the people who were signing on to Sacred Intimacy. I pecked Bob's cheek good-bye and left him to pack up his computer and papers. I walked the streets aimlessly, wondering how many others like me were out there. There must be a million Pams who would take comfort and find hope in the story of a kindred spirit. I just needed a way to spread the word without becoming the scandal du jour.

I'd just read a big article about the runaway blog train. Everyone was blogging about everything from food to office affairs. And so many were anonymous. It was perfect for me. My phone rang.

"Where are you?" Markus asked.

"On West 24th Street. Why?"

"Karmic coincidence. I love it. I'm coming to meet you right now. We're going shopping."

I checked the time. I had a few hours before I had to head home. Gavin was taking the boys to shoot some pool, and that translated to a pizza somewhere. I was off the hook for dinner.

"So what are we shopping for?"

"You need some adventures when we go to San Francisco. You have to have the right clothes." Markus was giddy with his plans. "First I am taking you to a dinner party to meet Joseph Kramer, the founder of Body Electric, Sacred Intimacy, and Sexological Body Work. You do have a little black dress, right? But it's time my goddess-in-training tried a session with a real pro dom. That's what we're shopping for. You need something tight and naughty. Honey, what I'm talking about ain't in your closet. I'll meet you at Purple Passion. You're about two blocks away."

I beat Markus to the store and waited outside. I looked in the window. I was not going in there alone. No way. I know what it's like to be a full-figured girl in the land of size 0. Humiliating didn't begin to touch it. Markus, lithe and slender and male, couldn't possibly understand what he was asking me to do. He didn't get that these getups were simply not made for me and my kind.

"So are you scared to go in without me?" Markus startled me.

"Maybe I am. They will have nothing for me in there. Worse, some skinny young thing will be helping me. This just isn't fun."

"Come on, princess! I've already told you, there is something for every shape. I think you might be surprised." With that, Markus put his arm around me and propelled me through the door. Behold Purple Passion.

As far as a shopping venue is concerned, Purple Passion was deceptive. The merchandising was a silent but insistent seduction. The first thing I bumped into was the fetish magazine section. Feet, bondage, spanking, big girls with big asses. I had no idea! Next to those were stacks of business cards of people who could help novices get comfortable with their fetishes. Workshops and individual sessions upon request. I walked past a display case filled with every kind of dildo and butt plug known to humankind. It was hypnotizing. Just a bit past that, hanging at eye level, were collars—beautiful rhinestone-encrusted ones, delicate ones, and some that looked exotic and slightly dangerous. They were right by the cash register. Now, that's what I call an impulse purchase. I saw things that I'd never seen before, like chairs that had nothing to do with sitting.

As I moved further away from the entrance, I encountered racks and racks of fetish clothing, floggers, paddles, more dildos, assorted masks, and other sex toys. Markus wasted no time. He rifled through the racks calling out brightly, "Look at this one." And I would stare hard, unable to see anything but a rubber dot. "Markus, I can't fit into that! Even if I could fit into that, no one would want to see me in it!" I mean, we're taking about the tiniest piece of latex anyone could manufacture.

This was every bit as awful as I had imagined, but Markus kept at it. One after another, he held up little smudges of leather, this one tied together with string, the next with silver chains. I frantically scanned for the exit sign.

"Hi! Can I help you guys?" The cheery, bold voice belonged to a large woman with an even bigger smile. Mistress Saleslady stood about five foot ten and was no lightweight. I felt positively dainty standing beside her. Maybe this would be okay. At least she would understand. Standing alongside her, a hope took root that this might not be such a humiliating experience. Sometimes I do believe that the universe gives us what we need.

"Yes! She's going to work with her first pro dom in San Francisco and needs a little something," Markus piped up.

Well, that was all out in the open. The thing was, Purple Passion was the kind of place where you could say that and no one would bat an eyelash.

In a small voice, I asked, "Do you have anything here that will fit me? Maybe with a little tummy support?"

She glanced over at Markus. I caught the "isn't she cute" exchange between them. Here I was standing in front of this plus-size girl asking if there was anything here to fit me! I blushed. I realized I was being rude. At the same moment part of me fretted that she was going to give me very loud directions to the only known plus-size fetish shop! I braced myself and my ego for the answer.

"Oh yes, honey," she said with a laugh. "I have things that'll look very hot on you! Don't you worry!"

With a muscular arm around my waist, Mistress Saleslady steered me into a dressing room in the back. "Get undressed and I'll bring you things to try on!"

Alrighty then. I knew when I was in the presence of a dominant. I stripped.

When she came back a few minutes later, she laced me into a black leather corset and a rubberized transparent skirt. I looked like a frilly twenty-pound sausage stuffed into a casing meant for half the meat. It was mortifying.

"Come out! Let me see!" Markus bellowed.

"Markus, *no!* I look silly."

Mistress Saleslady came in and pried my fingers from the wall. Grunting with the effort, she pulled me out of the dressing room, dragging me by the hand.

"Come on, honey. Let's show your friend," she panted.

"We'll take it." Markus decided after one look. "That's hot."

With each new outfit, I got bolder. I'd gather all the dignity I had, suck in my stomach as hard as I could, and walk out on my own for the public viewing.

"Turn around! Show me your butt!" Markus barked. "Try the rubber top with that! I love that!"

He was a goddamn drill sergeant! "Take that off! Put on the high boots! Oh, that is *sexy!*"

No one made fun of me. Why didn't I ever learn? After a while, through my nonstop nervous chattering about how fat I was, how I was not sure of this or that, I got into it, like a slightly inflated Versace model stomping down the runway.

It turned out that shopping with Markus and Mistress Saleslady was incredible! I started to feel sexy and hotter with each successive outfit. The exhibitionist in me enjoyed vamping for the two of them. Not once did anyone make a negative crack about my body. What I heard in one variation or another was, "Doesn't that look sexy on her?" and "That skirt would never look that good on me."

I loved my Mistress Saleslady. She only brought me things that she knew in her big-girl heart would work on my body. She meant business. I started to look in the mirror with kinder eyes. Could it be that my body didn't look half bad in these outfits? And if I looked at myself at just the right angle, I could say truthfully, I did look hot.

I wanted every single piece that worked for me. But boy oh boy, these items were not cheap! One could easily spend thousands of dollars. I cut my must-have pile in half, leaving behind a $400 old-fashioned silk corset that I wanted badly.

"Are you sure?" Mistress Saleslady asked, with a mournful little nudge. "Did you see yourself in that? Go look again."

"I can't. I have to accessorize, don't I?" I answered. (Translation: My kids have to eat.)

Markus led me to the accoutrements and I went on a minibinge. I got a leather paddle that was hard on one side, soft and furry on the other, and a cool collar with diamond accents, because I am a princess after all.

Three hours and $1,000 later, I rang up and checked out.

"I want to thank you from the bottom of my heart," I said to Mistress Saleslady. I was slightly teary but had a big smile plastered on my face.

She shook my hand and grinned back. I could see that both she and Markus were exhausted. I admit it, I'm a handful.

We left the store, loaded down like packhorses, and stepped into the last rays of a brilliant sunset. Markus stopped me in the street and gave me one of his piercing looks.

"So, Pamela, did you learn anything from this experience?"

Blech.

"Okay, Markus. I learned that if I trust and surrender, I can get out of my own way. I can get what I really want. I learned that I am not a great big huge whale and that there are lots of beautiful, fun, sexy things for me to wear. I learned that I can look and feel really, really sexy."

"Good, Grasshopper!" Markus chuckled. "You did great today!" He paused, scrutinizing me. "I think you're ready for what awaits in San Francisco. You're ready to surrender to your pro dom."

Moi? Trust and surrender are my middle names.

Chapter Thirty-One

Letting Gavin See

I KNEW THIS LEVEL of transparency was good for my marriage. I knew Gavin's willingness to do this was a testament to his love for me. I knew that this could be the beginning of a shift in our marriage. But it was as close to introducing your husband to your lover as one could possibly get without it actually being that. I fought back the frigid fingers of anxiety. Up until now Markus had been about me, my sexuality, and excavating my unknown, untapped desires. He had helped me make friends with my body again. Markus, my sexual healer, allowed me to discover that I had been hiding the true nature and depth of my libido and my human potential. It took months of work for me to figure out that I wasn't doomed to a life of low or no sexual interest and a crappy self-image. I wanted all the women in my life to know what was possible. So far, all I'd done was tell them about Sacred Intimacy. But none of them had taken a bite of the apple yet. On the other hand, sharing a Markus session with Gavin meant taking a leap into "us" and "our" sexuality. That was a different universe. I was afraid that whatever control I'd won over my life might be lost the minute Gavin shook Markus's hand. Plus, the Tiger was so good-looking that I worried it might freak Gavin out. I felt vulnerable. I was either the bravest woman on the face of the earth or completely mad.

I think Gavin felt as scared as I did. We tacitly agreed to avoid any conversation about the session beyond the basics of date, time, and place. We didn't know what to say. We had no idea what might happen. So we both treated it as if it were happening to somebody else.

But there we were, riding the elevator to Markus's apartment. It was an excruciating two minutes of meaningful looks and dense silence.

"Hello, Mr. and Mrs! Welcome!" Markus opened the door. In his sarong du jour, with bare chest and banging coral beads, he was quite the contrast to my Mister in his Top-Siders and Dockers. The men greeted each other with polite handshakes. Gavin and I shed sweaters and went right to the famous talk-therapy area. Markus had thoughtfully arranged three chairs and provided cold beer. Despite the prenoon hour, Gavin popped one and settled back with a "Thanks, man."

"I know we're all feeling nervous," Markus said. "This is a new, big step. So let's do a meditation and breathing exercise to begin, just to center ourselves."

I snuck a glance at my husband, the pragmatic antithesis of a New Age guy. He had on his "I'm trying so hard" face. I was sure I had on my "I want to vomit" face.

"What brings you here today?"

Did Markus take his meds this morning? What brings us here?

Gavin surprised me by jumping right in.

"Pam has been really interested in all of this Sacred Sexuality stuff. She told me that she likes spanking and you know how to do it. I don't know anything about that, but I offered to try. She seemed reluctant without my getting some training, so she suggested we come here. I figured I could learn how to spank. And maybe some other things, too. I don't know if this is for me, but I love her."

Gavin was talking more at one time than I could ever remember. "Pammy's been honest with me about her activities. I don't know all the details. I don't know if I want all the details. But I know that she's really happy and that this has been good for her."

He paused to catch the next thought. "In many ways it's been good for our marriage, too. She goes out of her way these days to make me happy. I've noticed that we don't fight nearly as much. And if we do fight, she doesn't throw in the kitchen sink. She doesn't seem to need to anymore. I know that her time with you has . . . with this work has . . . "

Gavin stumbled a little. I gave him a supportive nod. "I want her to stay happy. If I can be a part of this in any way, I am willing to explore it. She's way ahead of me, but I'm open."

I was staring at Gavin. That was some soliloquy. I couldn't believe it. Who was this guy?

"Pam, are you doing okay?" Markus looked at me.

I was sitting in what had been my private space with Markus. Now Gavin was in it, too. I felt all hot and sweaty. It wasn't sexy. I couldn't get past the fact that I was doing what I swore I'd never do from the very beginning. I was bringing my worlds together. Then again, I never expected this to become my passion, my mission. Didn't my husband deserve to be a part of it? Besides, Markus was convinced that this was the right thing to do. But I wasn't sure I liked being officially secretless. Why couldn't I have taken up bridge?

"I'm okay. I'm just feeling a little shaky about all of this."

Gavin looked as cool and collected as I'd ever seen him. So did Markus. Apparently I was the only one having a stroke.

"Gavin, how would you feel if I demonstrated a touching exercise on Pam?"

"Sure! Why not. Have at her," Gavin chirpily responded, swigging his beer.

My mouth opened and closed like a bass caught in a net.

"Pam?" Markus turned his stare on me. "How about you?"

I was too dumbfounded to do anything other than gasp. I hadn't thought about what this would actually look like. I somehow never thought that it would really happen.

Markus left the room for a minute and, like Pavlov's dogs drooling, I started to undress. When the Tiger left the room it was always my cue to strip. Now it was beyond weird. My God, my husband was here. I was embarrassed and anxious, but I told myself not to think about it.

"Pam! What are you doing?" Markus walked back in and stared, astonished at my nude body.

I watched the red rise from my feet to my chest.

"You said that we were going to do a touching exercise. I thought I was supposed to get undressed." I was so mortified that I wanted to cry.

"Well, Pam, that's fine. But we could have done this with your clothes on."

If I could have fled that apartment, I would have run stark naked down eleven flights of stairs in record time.

I tried to center myself with a deep breath. I asked myself to surrender to this moment.

With both of us standing in front of Gavin, Markus began.

"Notice that I hold her in my gaze, Gavin."

I was staring back, but my eyes were filled with tears. This was so much for me. I had voluntarily and unnecessarily stripped down in front of my husband and my sexual healer. I was about to be touched in front of my beloved by a man with whom I had an unusual and extremely intimate relationship. It was one thing to tell Gavin about this. It was quite another to have him watching from a front-row seat.

Markus included Gavin in everything, explaining every touch. I heard it all from a million miles away.

"Notice how she surrenders into my arms," Markus said as he pulled me close, running his hands along my flanks and over my breasts. My body instinctively responded and a moan escaped my lips. All this evidence laid out for Gavin put me over the edge. Thankfully, the blood rushing in my ears dimmed the voices. I closed my eyes and willed myself into an erotic trance.

Markus was teaching Gavin as he touched me. I sighed. I moved. I went where Markus took me. I floated until Markus moored me back into the moment.

"How are you doing, princess?" Markus asked, bringing me back to earth.

I slowly opened my eyes and the first thing I saw was Gavin. I burst into tears. He stood up and held me.

"Oh God, Gavin. I don't know. I feel like I let you see me just now. All of me. The way I really am. For the first time in I don't know how long, one hundred years? And I felt truly seen by you."

Gavin took my face and held it in his hands. He looked directly into my eyes. "I know. I know. I understand. Thank you. You are beautiful."

And then I kissed Gavin, open, on the mouth, the way that I hadn't in decades. It was so good to be in his arms.

While we hugged, Markus set up the massage table with pillows arranged to mimic the human form, putting out floggers of every description.

"Floggers, Markus?" I asked sotto voce. "My playbook was about spanking, not this."

"Why so coy, honey?" the Tiger answered. "I thought we would have a buffet. You love buffets."

Unfazed, Gavin shuffled over to the table for Flogging for Beginners. The Tiger gave him the dos and don'ts. "You must always avoid the spine," Markus said. Gavin looked worried. But the teacher kept on teaching, giving my husband the lowdown on how to use power and surrender in sexual play. After what felt like hours, Gavin got the chance to practice on the pillows. He had surprisingly good aim and handled the flogger with ease.

"Your sailorman likes the leather. Aren't you the lucky Mrs." I hated Markus.

I watched all of this in nervous anticipation. I was very unclear about what was going to happen next, but I was pretty sure it involved my ass up on the table for "Amateur Jack" to take a whack at.

"Well, Pamela, how would you feel about having two beautiful men work on your body for a little while?"

Markus's deep ocean eyes looked into mine, checking in with me to see if we were okay. My eyes welled up again and I nodded. This was so much for me, to be intimate with both of them when each knew me so differently and so thoroughly. It was hard to look at Markus with Gavin right there. I felt exposed. I kept waiting for some kind of negative reaction from Gavin as he witnessed the intimacy between me and Markus.

"Let's start with you on your tummy, sweetie," Markus said.

I was glad to hop up on the table, lie down, and close my eyes. It was a bit of the escape I was looking for.

"I'll stand by her head for a little while, Gavin, while you begin to work on the rest of her body." Markus moved to my head and I felt his hands run through my hair. "She loves to have her hair played with. Do you know that? When she's all hot and bothered, she really enjoys having her hair tugged on a little bit," he said, giving a pull.

Oh God. He is telling Gavin about what I like! I couldn't

imagine how that would go over. I kept worrying Gavin was wondering, *How does he know that?*

I knew that Gavin understood that Markus did erotic and sensual touch on my body. We just hadn't discussed many of the details. Now Gavin was learning the closeness of my relationship with Markus. It was hard to breathe.

Instead of strangling me and throwing Markus off the terrace, Gavin started to run his hands over my body. His hands were very calm. They didn't feel upset or angry. I relaxed as Gavin gently massaged me while Markus rubbed my head and stroked my hair.

The music started to change to a more pulsing beat and the men began to pick up the energy with their touch. It became more erotic. They were moving from calming the frightened goddess to waking her up. I began to move under their touch. Markus continued to coach Gavin and make suggestions as they traveled my body's terrain together.

Then I felt the swish and thwack of the flogger hit my back. Gavin wasn't shy with the whip. Perhaps he was enjoying this a bit too much. I grinned to myself.

He played with the flogger, using deep and light touch. My body responded. I moved to his ministrations. While Gavin was flogging me, Markus spanked and teased the rest of my body. I was awash with touch and sensation. Gasping and moaning, bouncing and wiggling, pure physical sensation took me totally out of my head. I was shameless. Markus said, "We might have to tie her up if she doesn't stop moving so much!"

Nothing else mattered but the touch that crashed and washed over me.

A torrent of rapid flogging rained down. Gavin and Markus were flogging me in tandem! "Notice she is not saying 'red'! Notice there hasn't even been a 'yellow' yet. That is important to notice!"

Markus coached. "Look at her body. Her ass is reaching for more. Pay attention to body cues!"

I felt laughter bubble up from some place inside of me. I was on a great big ride and it was so much fun! I felt like a wild woman!

"Let's have your beautiful wife turn over now."

Four hands gently assisted me in rolling over onto my back. My husband leaned down and kissed me on my mouth. "You are such a great big slut," he murmured lightheartedly. And Markus didn't skip a beat! "Your wife? A slut? Your wife is a huge touch pig."

I was so glad that the men could bond over my endless desire for more! Markus applied scented cream to my skin. My opera of moaning moved into the second act.

Those men collaborated in bringing me to five climaxes. I was beginning to worry about infarcting right there. I couldn't catch my breath. "Red . . . red . . . no more . . . please . . . I can't. . . . "

"The Goddess of More is complete? Could that be true?" Markus teased.

Gavin was kissing my mouth, my hair, all of me. I felt so loved. Markus left the room. Gavin gathered me up in his arms and held me. "I think I would like to take you to lunch now and buy you a big steak and a dirty martini. Would you like that, honey?"

I looked, blurry-eyed, at the clock. Oh my God, we had been here for well over four hours! I was starving. I eased myself off the table, and Gavin watched me dress.

We thanked Markus and headed out the door. With Markus's help we had created a new passage in our marriage. What would we do with it? Unclear. But what was clear was that Gavin and I loved each other and wanted to grow old together.

Markus told me later that he watched us walk to our car from his terrace. "My heart grew two sizes seeing you hand in hand, strolling down the street."

Chapter Thirty-Two

MOTHERLOAD

WE WERE BOTH lost in thought on the drive back to the Bronx. We went to the old Irish pub on Riverdale Avenue, the one place we knew we could find a good steak and decent drinks without breaking the bank. We sat facing each other in an old, worn leather booth and ordered without glancing at the menu. Gavin reached over and held my hands, like he always did.

"So, what do you think?" I asked, a little tentative.

"I feel better knowing what's going on. The reality of it doesn't threaten me like I was afraid it might," he said. "It was fun."

"And . . . "

"I'm sorry you got embarrassed getting naked, but I'm glad you did it. I don't think I would have understood what this means for you if you hadn't taken off your clothes."

"Well, would you like to have another session? Maybe the next time you could get on the table and really experience what I do."

"Uh, ah, Pammy, I love you. You know I do. But no. I get why you go, I love that we did this together. But honestly, this isn't for me."

He watched me deflate. "But it went so well. What's the problem?" I heard a plaintive whine in my voice.

"There is no problem, honey. I don't force you to play pool. I can't get you to set foot on a sailboat. And it's okay. But now I know I'm right about myself. It's better for me if my fantasies stay in my head. The only exploring I want to do is in our bed or in my dreams. It's who I am."

I tried to keep my disappointment from flooding the T-bone platter. In some way, I was back to where I started—this was about me and only me. But then again, my marriage proved sound enough to survive a four-handed flogging. Gavin was content to let me be and not shut me down. There was a lot of comfort in that.

Well, if he is this cool with it, I thought, *why not?* He looked peaceful enough.

"You know, I've been thinking," I said.

The color drained from Gavin's face. He knocked back the rest of his whiskey and waited for my next "throw us into chaos" idea.

"How would you feel if I wrote about my experiences?" There was something seriously wrong with me.

"What do you mean? You're not thinking about a book, are you? With your name? Your real name?"

My poor honey. "No. Relax. I was thinking more along the lines of a blog. It would be anonymous. You know how to do that, don't you, Gavin? You could help keep me protected in the blogosphere? You're so good at that high-tech sort of thing. Practically a genius."

For once, Gavin was speechless.

A few loaded minutes passed while he fortified himself with another whiskey. Guess I was the designated driver.

"Pammy, do you know what you're doing? Anonymity is pretty flimsy. Anyone could pierce that veil if they wanted to. I know you're not going to be able to keep your mouth shut about it. I don't think it's a good idea for you to put yourself out there like that."

"I want to." I surprised myself with my vehemence. "I need to put this work—not myself—out there. You see how amazing it can be, how it has transformed me. I have so much to say. It heals me. Everyone should know Sacred Intimacy is a possibility."

His shoulders sagged in resignation. "This is yet another oil spill about to happen, isn't it? There's no way to put a cap on you."

I promised him there'd be no environmental disaster if he'd steer the technology.

The next morning, "The Riverdale Goddess: The Very Unusual Adventures of a Not So Ordinary Riverdale Housewife" was born.

Like every novice blogger, I had no clue if anyone was reading. But I got up every morning at five a.m., made coffee, and wrote down everything that had happened over the past year—give or take. I gave up each memory and posted it raw. I made up my mind not to edit or pretend I was something I wasn't. Within days, I got my first comments. Three weeks in, I had a following. They were articulate, supportive, judgment-free, opinionated, male and female, gay and straight, married, single, and separated. I was writing my story and people related. They identified with me. I identified with them. How they found me, I didn't know. But the Riverdale Goddess hit a nerve and had a community. I was flying.

Gavin was right. I couldn't shut up. I just had to tell my mother.

Even at this age, my mother was a sensual animal. She wore her SEXY GRANDMA charm necklace instead of a MedicAlert. In her younger days, she was the Brooklyn-born Marilyn Monroe of Great Neck, Long Island. These days, she was busy being a girlfriend. Everybody's girlfriend. She hated it if she had even an inkling that my friends knew something about my sister or me that she didn't.

She'd been circling around me, smelling the sauce. "Where are *you* off to in that 'look at me' outfit? You're out all the time. I hope Gavin doesn't mind."

I knew she could take my discoveries in stride. But still, she was my mother. I had to manage the situation, control the environment, put a time limit on it. I took her to the Cheesecake Factory for lunch, the way I did every few weeks.

"Mom, you remember Markus, right? My life coach? He's the cute blond guy you met at my house. Remember? He was picking up some folding chairs for a group he was running."

"Of course, Pammy. He's a very lovely man. It's nice that you can have a male friend and Gavin doesn't mind. I suppose it doesn't hurt that he's gay."

She had no idea.

"Listen, Mom. Don't interrupt. Markus is more than my life coach. He's also a sexologist."

Mom's eyes popped and I could feel her winding up. I forged ahead before she could say a thing.

"He is like a sex therapist. I've worked with him for almost a year now and it's changed my life." Well done. The first part was out.

"Ha! I *knew* something was going on," she squealed. "I could just feel it! All of this 'goddess this, goddess that' talk!" Mom inhaled and broadsided me. "So you have sex with him?"

I actually bristled. I have no idea why. "No, Mother. There is *no* sexual intercourse or oral sex. Ever. Markus isn't a sexual surrogate; he's not an escort or a prostitute. Not that there's anything wrong with that. He's a certified sexologist and something called a Sacred Intimate. He works with people using sexual energy to help them heal their life issues."

She looked puzzled, but not disgusted. So I kept going.

"Usually we talk first. We talk about what's going on in my

life—you know, things with Gavin, the boys, work. Then he gives me a sensual massage."

My mother raised an eyebrow. "So *that's* what we are calling it now? A 'massage'?"

We both burst out laughing. Once I caught my breath, I continued down the path of enlightenment.

"It's so hard to explain the power of this work, Mom. But I don't binge on food anymore. I don't feel ashamed of my body. Most of the time. You know that's been an issue forever. In many ways, Markus and some of the other therapists that I have worked with have saved my life. It's been incredible."

"You mean there are others?"

Emotion grabbed me by the throat. My eyes welled. She saw my expression, reached out her hand, and gave my shoulder a comforting rub.

"Then you keep doing it," she said, looking straight at me.

She grew quiet for a few minutes. I was on tenterhooks.

"Tell me, how is Gavin with all of this? That Markus is very handsome."

"Actually, Mom, Gavin is fine. Gavin wants to stay married and so do I. He knows that I need to explore my sexuality in a way that I can't with him. We're trying. He wants me to be happy. He likes Markus and trusts him. We've even done a couples session. So he knows what's what. He knows there are boundaries, so he feels safe about me working with Markus and with me doing workshops."

"Workshops? You go to workshops?"

"Uh-huh. I love them. There's an entire community of people out there who've combined sexuality with spirituality. There are always instructors around. It's group learning and exploration. And it's fun. It's safe. I promise you that I am safe."

How many times could I say "safe" in one conversation?

Mom mulled this over for a few beats, then asked, "Are you worried about becoming attached to Markus? If I was doing what you were doing with that sexy man, I think I would become attached."

She's so perceptive she made me want to weep. Or scream.

"Well, honestly, I *am* attached to Markus. We've become good friends. But he's my Sacred Intimate first—my teacher and caregiver. We're clear about that. But we are close and I do love him. Just not in that way. Which would be impossible anyway. Like you said, he's gay. I'd never even be in the game."

"All right. Good. You know what you're doing. You're open with Gavin, which I'm relieved about, you know. And you look great. Who else knows?"

"A lot of people." I ticked off the names. She was incredulous and a little jealous.

"You mean I'm the last one to know? How could you do that to me?"

"For God's sakes, Mother. You're my mother. Can you please cut me some slack?"

"So you told everybody? Vicki? Beth? Everyone?"

"Yes, Mother. Everybody. I took out an ad in the *Times* just this week. And Mom, there's something else. I'm writing a blog. Every day. It's anonymous but honest. Are you embarrassed?"

"Me? Embarrassed? I think it's great!" She grew thoughtful. "You know, Pammy, I don't know why you don't put your name on it. Why not? There's nothing to hide. Everyone's talking about sex. You can do it better than that Carrie Bradshaw person." Of course, Carrie Bradshaw was pure fiction, but this was a start.

Chapter Thirty-Three

The Kinky Daughter and the Jewish Mother

Open, honest living suited me just fine. I was waking up more relaxed and managing to get through my frenzied days with unfamiliar calm. This day was pretty typical, except for the little ripples of excitement that came over me whenever I thought about the upcoming trip. My blog was done by the crack of dawn. I'd conducted a virtual staff meeting, driven Andrew back to his Manhattan college dorm, and taken an hour to have my hair done—I wanted to look gorgeous for my first tryst with a pro dom. Then, before heading back to Riverdale, I made a downtown detour to pick up smoked fish and bagels at *the* place for appetizers, Russ & Daughters. When I got home I'd be a "good daughter," put on a pot of coffee, and invite my mother over for a late brunch.

I hadn't done that in a long time and I felt the pangs of guilt. What with San Francisco only a few days away, I had precious little time in my schedule. But, she is my mother. Sometimes I had no patience for her. But today I felt like I could do it! I felt strong!

Coffee brewed, bagels in the oven. Enter Mom!

"I'll have half a bagel and bring the other half home. With the lox," she said, as if I didn't know. While I prepared her doggie bag we put on *Oprah* and half-watched Tom Cruise fall apart on national TV. The whole time my mother talked a blue streak.

"Pam, this belly lox is unbelievable. That Cruise fella is meshuga! Don't you think so? I mean, look at him. Did I tell you I'm planning a trip to Costa Rica with the girls? How is Gavin *really* doing with your whole new life?"

She waited for a reaction. She didn't get one. I puttered around the apartment, keeping my hands from criminal activity. I dusted, straightened, put away clean undies in my lingerie drawer.

"Hey! Do you want to see my sexy clothing?" It was out of my mouth before I knew it. A spontaneous emission. "Do you want to see the other side of your homemaker daughter up close and personal?"

"Really? What fun! Will you model them for me?"

Without hesitation, I pulled on my black stockings and high black boots. What the hell. I was giving my mother an erotic-lingerie fashion show!

"Oh my God!" Mom shrieked. "Look at that! The string goes right through your vagina! That is *so* sexy! Does it bother you? You know your father didn't like that I wore cotton lollipop panties. Who knew what else there was to wear? But apparently *he* knew, that bastard." A wry snicker. "What else have you got in there?"

I put on my new rhinestone bra that opened in the front to reveal my breasts.

"You know your breasts need support at all times," my mother commented. "You know that, right?"

"What are you saying, Mom? That my breasts are sagging?"

"No. I'm not saying that."

Yes she was.

"Mom, my nipples do not point down. They point straight

ahead or even up a little. I have full breasts. This is how they sit on my body. I am a C- or D-cup, for heaven's sake!"

I pulled my breasts up to an unnatural angle. "Do they look normal to you if I do that?" I threw down the challenge.

I waited while my mother carefully considered the aesthetics of my full, weighty boobs in a gravity-defying position.

"No . . . they don't, Pammy," she finally answered. "You're right. We're so used to seeing surgically enhanced breasts I think, even at my age, I forget what's natural. I don't know why any breasts around your size should stick out like balloons. It's sick. But you do know that you should always wear support, Pammy. You need to protect the muscles. That way they won't sag."

No good, I'm now feeling defensive about my breasts. "Mom, I always wear a bra."

"Even around the house?"

"Mom, around the house I wear a yoga top with a built-in bra. Okay?"

She looked at me in my outfit the way a kosher butcher might eye a brisket for the holidays.

"It's amazing to me how good your legs look. You had these fat *pulkies* before. Your legs look amazingly firm now." How many times was she going to say that she was amazed? "It's too bad about your C-section. You used to have such a perfectly flat tummy. They did that to me, too, those damn doctors. I guess you could have that fixed if you wanted to. I like this G-string better than that one because, you know, it covers you a little there, you know, where the scar is."

Self-conscious and a tad murderous, I defaulted into sex-enlightened mode. "Mom, one of the things that has been good for me in my explorations and workshops is that I get to see all kinds of bodies. Very few of them are flawless. And let me tell you, there are imperfect *thin* bodies, too. Sometimes, Mother, being too thin can be odd-looking. People have all kinds of scars, or hair or no hair. Breasts come in all sizes. So do cocks and balls. Some men have balls that hang to their knees and they're swollen like grapefruits! I have seen three-hundred-pound women flaunting it and being worshipped. I mean it, Mom, worshipped. Every big, fat fold of flesh.

"That's been liberating. I know that I have a little lower tummy—it has gotten so much better, or didn't you notice? I'm evenly proportioned. I'm fit. God, Mom, I'm five years away from fifty! This body has birthed children and nursed them. It's gained seventy pounds and lost thirty. It works hard!

"I'm finally okay with not being perfect. No one's perfect. Perfection is bullshit and too many people put their lives on hold waiting until they reach their ideal. It never happens. I'm not waiting any more. I look sexy and feel very hot right now!"

I had to admit it, my mother's understanding and approval were core to me. I needed her to accept me exactly the way I was. I wanted her to tell me that I looked great with thirty pounds gone. I needed her reassurance that I wasn't making a fool out of myself in my little costumes.

"Well," she said appraisingly, "you look amazingly good." There was that word again. "And you're right. There are all kinds of bodies. And if you want surgery, you can have a tummy tuck later."

Oh God . . . she's honest! Perhaps I should get a gun now and put myself out of my misery. Yet for Mom and me, we were doing great.

She loved my leather vest and my see-through skirt. I showed her how I could unveil myself in layers. She was all smiles.

"Love that little chain-bra thing! I'm so glad that I didn't go to bridge class! This is so much more fun. Look at what I would have missed! Thank you. And, you know, you really *do* look great. And I'm sorry that I said anything about your breasts. They are beautiful. You really have *my* breasts, you know, and I'm just looking out for them.

"And this spanking thing! I try not to think about that! You know, you were never spanked much as a child. I really don't understand *that* at all!"

Mom paused to take us both in. She glanced down at her coordinated Talbots turquoise and neon green jogging suit ("Perfect for Florida!") and me in my thigh-high leather boots and not much else. "Honey, you must put this in your blog. Okay? Trust me. Everyone's gonna love it."

Chapter Thirty-Four

And Now for Something Completely Different

The downside of transparency was that every morning my mother called to review the blog. After weeks of anticipation, I was in a packing frenzy trying to cram every Purple Passion item into two mingy bags, and not having much success. I was late picking up Markus for the flight to San Francisco. Beth was already at the airport. She called every five minutes. "Where are you? The frigging plane is gonna take off without us. Get your ass in gear."

I popped a Xanax. Flying made me crazy. So did Beth. Call-waiting beeps interrupted her harangue. For once I was glad to see my mother's number pop up.

"Gavin's driving us to the airport as soon as I'm ready. I gotta go."

"I can't read this at night. I get too excited!" she shrieked.

"Mom! I can't really talk now. I'm packing. I'm late. I have to get to the airport. And you know how much I love flying." Silence. "Okay, Mom, what can't you read at night?"

"Were you really with that Rock in New Mexico? That's where you were? You told me it was yoga." She was getting increasingly shrill. "What's with the wind and the air and the earth? You were a dancing fire? Was it shooting out from between your legs? I *knew* you weren't at a yoga place. You never do yoga. And what's the big mystery about a G-spot? I know just where to find mine. Have for years."

"Um-hmm. That's great, Mom. Good for you." I was not nearly as excited by this revelation as she was. Maybe the drugs were finally kicking in. "Anything else, Mom?"

"Did you read *New York Magazine* this week? They had a big piece on anal sex! They even showed a picture of an anus! I'm starting to think that maybe you are not as avant-garde as you think!"

She never failed to wear me down. Since I let her in on my blog, she insisted on giving me minute-by-minute critiques and media briefings. It was like X-rated TiVo run amok.

Honestly, how many people can say that their mothers called up with anal sex updates. This would put most mortals into long-term therapy! Oh wait. I *was* in long-term therapy.

"I'm on it. Don't you worry. I got anal sex covered," I said, and slammed down the phone.

There was not a minute to spare. Gavin had the car waiting in front. I edged a neighbor out of the elevator with my bags and ran to the car. I was hardly buckled in before Gavin floored it. We scooped up Markus and made it through airport security just before the gate closed. Markus, Beth, and I didn't exchange a word until we were wedged together in human-cargo class. Before Beth could let me have it for cutting it so close, my phone went off.

"You just had to tell Mom, didn't you."

Didn't anyone in my family say hello? I laughed.

"Of course I did. I'm the goddess of transparent living. You would not believe the fabulous leather corset I bought. I'm letting you in on my big secret, Vic. I'm going to do my first session with a real, honest-to-goodness pro dom."

"Oh God," Vicki groaned. "Are you going to blog about that, too? Mom just called me, hysterical. She couldn't understand why you would masturbate in a circle. She was really confused by that. Frankly, me too. And now you're going to go see a professional what?"

Sharing this part of my life with my mom and big sister had turned into a weekly smackdown. They tag-teamed me. I mean, my blog wasn't supposed to be this interactive.

"Passengers, please prepare for takeoff."

"Gotta go, Vic."

We landed at SFO and I was sky-high with excited anticipation. I love San Francisco. I love the people. I love the hills. I love dim sum in Chinatown. I love Japantown and the sushi boat bars. I loved that I was heading into unknown territory with Beth by my side and the Tiger's safety net there to catch me.

I arrived in that gorgeous city floating on a silver-rimmed cloud.

Beth looked like she was still airborne from her birthday session with Markus a few weeks ago. Once she calmed down, she spent the entire flight leaning over to whisper things to me. "Does he wear the leather gloves with you? Omigod, he's so hot. I don't know how you drive home after your sessions. I almost drove into a tree after mine. You know, he gave me the leather gloves because I loved them so much."

Wait a minute, now. She got the leather gloves after one session? I've been seeing him for a year and she gets the gloves and I get a bento box? I looked at Markus sleeping like a baby next to me. I wanted to punch him. It takes a strong woman to share her Sacred Intimate, I was learning. It was as if Markus's studio had a revolving door and all of a sudden, my friends were going through. The green-eyed monster had paid a visit or two. But it was so totally worth it. Just thinking about seeing Bitsy's face when I scooped her up after her first Tiger time, like I promised I would, was enough. Markus propped her up as he walked her from his building to my car, pouring her into the passenger seat. Her cheeks were flushed. I knew that face. It could have been mine. It was the face of a woman who had just spent a good deal of time lost in pleasure. There was no makeup. She didn't need any. It's what a woman became after she got acquainted with her desire. I felt pure joy for her.

"It was better than red velvet cake," she sighed, and burst into giggles. "Oh my God! Pamela! OMG! I want more! And more! And more! And more!"

"I know, Bits. We're so starved for this, we don't even know we're hungry."

With her eyes as big as saucers, she said, "He asked me about my desires! It stopped me dead, Pammy. *My* desires? Really? No one ever asked me about my desires before. I didn't know what to say. I wasn't even sure that I knew what they were! But I knew I had them—and I wanted to explore them. I don't think I can stop now. I don't want to stop. I think I've come alive again."

Shameless. Delicious. Fabulous. So what if I got jealous once in a while.

Once we collected our bags, we loaded ourselves into a cab. The Golden Gate Bridge filled me with optimism. I fell under the spell of the Queen Anne Hotel. With its deep red walls and velvet sofas, it looked like an old Victorian bordello. And I mean that in a good way. Every day at four p.m., the management put out no-name sherry and butter cookies. Markus wouldn't let me have any. Apparently that wasn't part of my new lifestyle, but I adored that they were offered. I loved that the Queen Anne billed itself as haunted and that a silly ghost tour started at our hotel. I loved that it was walking distance to everything. I spent the next two days wandering the city, fantasizing about using the new black leather corset I had bought on the East Coast, wondering how the hell I was ever going to get into it.

There was something daunting about working with a pro dom and a complete stranger, to boot. I wanted to look the part. The man that Markus found for me wasn't what I had expected. Dark Knight—or DK, as I thought of him—was a painter with a PhD in the fine arts. He was featured in a bunch of articles and even a documentary about the use of sexual energy and healing. He was intriguing. I looked at his pictures and fell for his blue, blue eyes.

I was supposed to call when I landed to check in with him and have an initial intake conversation. His phone rang and my brain boiled with twitchy thoughts. It felt too scary. If it had been someone from any of my workshops, I'd feel safe enough to dive in. I mean, it's possible that my hands would be tied. And my feet! If he wasn't totally honorable, I'd be in deep shit.

I hung up before he answered. I needed a plan in order to speak with him. Maybe Markus could be part of the session. That'd give me a safety net. I pulled up DK's photo again and studied it carefully. I was ready for voice contact. I dialed.

"Hello, this is Dark Knight." I thought it was his answering machine, but it was the man himself.

"Hi, Dark Knight. It's Pamela. I'm the one visiting from New York. Markus referred me. And I have a black corset with nowhere to go! So I'm looking forward to our session. I'm thinking that I'd like to bring Markus—the Tantric Tiger—to co-top me in the session."

Nerves had turned me into a nonstop talking machine. DK laughed. He had a lovely deep laugh.

"Pamela, I'm more than willing to work with you. But I don't eat family style."

I interrupted. "I'm a little scared. I've never done anything like this before. . . . "

"I'm unclear how Markus's presence would help with that. I need to build intimacy with you," he explained. "If I am not alone with you, I'm not sure that would happen. You will need to connect with me in session. If Markus is there, it will change the energy."

Wow. He was strong. He was hot. It gave my heart a little jump. This man wasn't willing to share the stage. Or me. I liked that. It actually made me want to work with DK more. A man in his power—a man willing to say no. It turned me on. Well, okay, then, maybe Markus would walk me there.

I booked for three hours. And I still couldn't stop the mouth machine. I let DK know that outside of sessions with Markus, I had little experience with dominance and submission. DK asked me a few more questions about my expectations.

"What do you like?" he probed.

"Well, you should know I'm not a pain freak. Black and blue aren't my colors," I told him with a lightness I didn't feel.

"Yes, now I know what you don't like. What do you like?" He was focused, I'll give him that.

"Um, I do like intensity of sensation. I like the power dynamics of surrendering to a strong male energy." Then, talking through my embarrassment, I added, "I enjoy spanking. I do like my bottom."

To that, DK responded, "That's good. We will put your bottom to good use, then!"

This man started the session before we even met in person. Now, *that* was some top energy.

I completely forgot that Markus could hear me. The Tiger's sniggering came through the wall. "You told DK that you were a beginner?" Markus burst into full belly laughs. "This filly has been trotted out of the stall a few times!"

I walked into his room and tackled him. I started laughing, too. "Okay, okay. But you gotta admit this is different. He's a pro, not a fellow student in a supervised workshop."

I did say I needed adventure. I had a hunch this would be everything I wanted. Maybe more.

Chapter Thirty-Five

Power, Surrender, and Intimacy: The Dark Knight

Markus helped lace me into my corset with strong hands and potent compliments. Beth sat on the bed watching my transformation. "That corset is so sexy, I'd do you. Markus, pull it tighter. She can still breathe."

If I wasn't mistaken, a small undercurrent of proprietorship ran through both of them. I was Markus's work in progress, and he was sending me off to a master. In this moment, he was my chivalrous accomplice. But it was Beth that got to me. It was one of the few times in our long history of often unspoken competitiveness that she had shown me loving encouragement free of jealousy. She told me I was hot and I believed her.

Markus left nothing to chance. "Don't forget a change of clothes for after your session. We're not taking you to dinner looking like that. Even if it is San Francisco and you look fabulous!"

"Ah c'mon," Beth said. "Let's take her to dinner looking just like that. Even better, let's go to a Nob Hill four-star for drinks with Pam all collared and leashed. Anyone got a ball gag?"

"Oh, will you both shut up. I'm a wreck as it is." I was having enough trouble filling my lungs with my waist reduced to half its size and my rib cage cinching my organs. "I'm gonna pass out, Markus!"

"Relax, you'll get used to it."

Beth didn't look so sure. "Can you walk in those things?" she asked, studying my black patent-leather four-inch platform stilettos.

"She'll be fine." Markus, the voice of experience, wrapped my black cloak around me like a shield and steadied me with a strong hand. Beth pulled up my "stay-up" thigh-high, black seamed stockings. "Hard to believe it was only a few hours ago that six hundred people listened to you pontificate about the impact of environmental toxins on fertility. If they could only see you now."

I was too busy trying to not tip over to respond.

Markus carried my toy bag as I tottered after him down the stairs, through the Queen Anne's lobby, acutely aware of the jingle of the hardware on my leather bracelet cuffs, positive that everyone in the lobby could hear the racket, too. Beth waved good-bye from the landing. "Have fun."

Nobody gave me a second glance. God, I love San Francisco.

It was tricky getting into the cab without giving the driver an eyeful. The corset was clearly not designed for sitting. I kept seeing the driver's eyes in the rearview mirror, sneaking peeks into the backseat.

For the thousandth time I asked Markus if I looked as saucy, sexy, and fantastic as I felt. With infinite patience, Markus reassured me. I let my outfit set the mood and I daydreamed about the DK session. Not for long, though. It was only about three minutes before we arrived. Markus helped me maneuver from the cab to the elevator to DK's apartment door without breaking an ankle.

Looking exactly like his Web site photo, DK stood in the open door.

Markus and I greeted him. He showed both of us into his beautiful, light-filled space. An easel took center stage, and the walls were covered with his paintings. Markus kissed me good-bye. He looked straight at DK and said, "Take care of my girl."

Then he was gone.

DK was in loose-fitting khakis, more schoolteacher than pro dom. He was so casually dressed that I was suddenly self-conscious, certain that I looked overdone and silly. I didn't want to give up my cape and let DK see me in my outfit. Maybe I should have worn jeans. Maybe, maybe, maybe . . . too late now.

We did the required "get to know you" dance. DK talked about boundaries and safe words while I fidgeted with my seriously uncomfortable getup. I tugged on the cuffs and pulled up the corset. He stopped speaking business and out of the blue said, "You look great."

It was enough to relax me so that I could listen to his questions and answer them. He finished up by saying, "Remember, I may not be able to do certain things to you in session because of your boundaries. But I am the top. I may want you to touch my body. Do you understand that?"

Touch his body? I hadn't thought about that. But I nodded. My pulse thudded in my neck.

DK got up and led me into another room. It had a bed. And there was a sling! I'd never seen a sling before in person, only in porn movies. It was a two-foot-by-three-foot sheet of sturdy black leather suspended by chains from a heavy iron stand. There were stirrups! It was like an ob-gyn contraption gone mad. I steadied myself on a handy bookcase featuring a photo of a naked DK in full arabesque. Why did I find that comforting?

"Are you ready to accept my collar and surrender to me in this session?"

"Pardon?"

"Pamela, are you ready?" DK's voice grew markedly lower. Before my eyes, the polite professor morphed into the Dark Knight, a primitive and unapologetically masculine force. With the ground rules laid out and the green light from me, DK stopped asking for permission. I yielded. DK put a black leather collar around my neck and looked into my eyes. He was towering over me.

"Now we will stop having casual conversation," he said. "If you want to speak, you say, 'Please, sir, may I have a word?' Do you understand? You always address me as 'sir' or 'master.'"

I nodded.

"No words count here except your safe words. You can say 'no' or make any sounds that you like. But nothing ends the game unless you say 'red.' Do you understand?"

"Yes."

"Yes, what?"

Oh. "Yes, sir."

"Good girl. You learn fast. I like that. Look into my eyes."

He reached for my face and lifted my chin. I looked into DK's intense blue eyes. His stare vaporized any trace of my own masculine energy. My soft feminine core opened. The intimacy between us was instantaneous and intense. It shocked me. Who was this man who took possession of me and made me yearn to be his in that moment?

Standing cuffed and corseted, I knew with certainty that what I felt had nothing to do with the costume or the props. This wasn't theater. I wasn't playing a role. All that mattered, all that was real, was in that room.

"Good," he said, blindfolding me with a practiced hand. I was in darkness, tottering on impossible heels, struggling for balance.

He led me a few feet and put my hands around a metal pole. It was the sling. Oh God.

"You wait here. I have to change." He was changing? Into what? There was movement and I could hear chains rattling. My ears were alive to sound. He wrapped an arm around my waist to steady me and asked me to stand still. He slipped my feet out of my shoes. The relief!

"Thank you, sir."

I felt cuffs go around my ankles. DK spread my legs and secured them with chains. He lifted my arms and fastened my wrists with more chains. Apparently the sling had multiple uses.

I'd been nervous before, but not scared. This new reality sent a jolt of fear through me. "Sir, may I have a word."

"Yes."

"Sir, I am feeling scared."

"Good." He stroked my hair. "You look so luscious. If people could see you in that corset they would want to know what's underneath. I'm going to find that out very soon. It's all going to be for me."

Electricity was coursing through me.

DK's knee was between my legs as he lifted me off the ground. I was breathless. I was flying. He played with me. He toyed with me and flung me about. I went where he took me. It was rough and unnerving.

Then I was alone again and dangling from my cuffs.

I heard DK rummaging through something and then there was light. My blindfold was off. DK was holding me in his powerful gaze again. Once again, he surprised me. I saw loving kindness. I didn't expect such softness. His tender gaze told me I was safe. I may have been DK's doll for the session, but he had no intention of breaking his toys. I melted. Then the darkness of the blindfold returned.

DK started to play with the flogger. Light strokes caressed the front of me and then the back. He began to undress me. His hands loosened my corset releasing the ten-pound sausage stuffed into the casing meant for a five-pound dog. Any hint of humiliation about the avalanche of flesh was swept away by the sheer joy of breathing fully.

"Thank you, sir," I said softly. I couldn't believe I'd spent nearly $500 on a getup that I was thrilled to be out of.

Once I was naked, the intensity of the flogging increased. DK was playing with my edges. He broke up the sensations with words or gentle touch . . . a spank . . . or by lifting me completely off the ground with speed and ease. DK played with something sharp on my body. What was that?

He reassured me. "Don't worry, this pinwheel will not break your skin." Hell, I hadn't even considered that. Fear poked through for only a second before he released my wrists and ankles and led me, still blindfolded, to the bed. He had me lie down on my belly. I heard the chains. They made an incredible rattling. The unfamiliar sound was intimidating and sexy at the same time.

DK ran his hands over my body. I was in an altered state of pure desire. I felt like a vessel waiting to be filled. I was stripped of everything except the desire to be open. I felt the beginning of a spanking. DK paddled softly. I enjoyed it. My body was flirting with him, my bottom dancing. The paddling went on and on, the intensity rising and falling until I was gasping.

"You are going to take ten now," DK growled. "They are going to be hard. You will count each one and then ask for another. Do you understand?" I thought that they were already hard. I was scared again. "Yes, sir."

"Good."

DK used a leather paddle and the noise of it against my ass was as earth-shattering as the sensation it produced.

Whack!

"One! Thank you, sir. May I have another?" The impact of the paddle pushed the counting out of my body and through my mouth.

Whack!

"Two! Thank you, sir. May I have another?" I was doing this, why?

Oh God! Ten? I had never felt anything like this. This man was playing a very hard game. I was determined to play right along with him. I wasn't going to say 'red.' I was going to go for this ride and see where it took me.

Whack!

"Ow! Ahh!" I almost flew off the bed.

"Don't get behind on your counting," DK warned, low and menacing. Was this "top speak" for "if you screw up, there will be even more"?

"Three! *Three!* Thank you, sir, may I have another!"

Ten was especially hard. I yelped under DK's paddle. I didn't know I could hit those notes.

Then his hands were soft on my bottom. His voice was filled with sweet congratulations for my bravery. I was pretty impressed with myself, too. That was strong stuff. I thought I was at my limit when DK turned me over and caressed the front of me. He was everywhere. The blindfold came off.

I had a moment to take in more than his eyes. DK was rippled muscle bound by the black crisscross of a leather harness. His body was covered in twenty-two-karat gold piercings. I had never seen anything like them. They were beautiful against his skin. His earrings matched his nipple rings, which matched his belly button ring, which matched . . . oh my.

Breathe, Pamela! Breathe! DK was giving me so much pleasure. I felt like pliant dough under his hands.

"What would you enjoy, Pamela?" DK allowed a request. Facing my desires, speaking them aloud, was a dangerous minefield for me.

"May I go over your knee, sir?"

"Yes, Pamela. We can do that." DK went to work.

I was like the kid who rides a very, very scary roller coaster screaming her head off to make it stop and then nags to go again before the first ride is even over. Take me again, sir. Bring me *there* again, sir. Let me find my outer limits *again,* sir.

It felt so good to feel his warm, hard body against mine. I was dying to touch the gold rings. And then I was down again—and I rode. When I counted to ten again, when we got to that special place on DK's roller coaster, I discovered I'd traveled into what is known in the BD/SM underground as "sub space." I'd been in an erotic trance before with Markus, but never like this. I was so deep I wasn't sure how I'd ever resurface into my body.

DK flipped me over after spanking number two. He was beside me on the bed, brushing my hair away from my face with his fingers. "You look so beautiful right now," he whispered.

Sweet, that felt sweet to me. His touch, his words, and his eyes. I let myself simply be. I didn't need to know any more about him than I knew right then. His softness was as delicious as his strength. Maybe they were the same thing. The intimacy of that moment was as real as any between lovers. I savored the feelings that my Dark Knight summoned.

DK was indeed a master. He understood the dance of power and surrender and cultivated a partner in me. Perhaps it was the most important piece of all. My bottom was hot, my feminine core was fully awake. DK had possessed me in a way I covertly longed for but didn't believe existed outside romance novels. Yet there it was. DK was the wild buccaneer. I was the damsel who succumbed. It wasn't politically correct. It transcended thought. These feelings were primitive, from a time before words. Now that I'd bitten into the forbidden fruit, it was going to be really hard to leave the garden.

DK interrupted my reverie. "It's time to throw you into the sling!"

Of course it is.

Chapter Thirty-Six

Mistress Beth

I WOKE UP EARLY the next morning, all tingly and on a "bottom" rush. I slipped out of the room, careful not to wake Beth or Markus. They were still under the influence of the details and drinks I had lavished on them after they retrieved me from DK's place. I tiptoed down to the hotel lobby, psyched for what was now my pre-dawn blogging ritual. My online community of a few hundred was going to get a kick out of the day's post, "Goddess in Chains." I sank into a slightly worn armchair in front of the roaring fire that made the Queen Anne sitting room toasty. The computer booted up and I began. Between sips of my first cup of coffee, I wrote about every single Dark Knight second. I got myself excited all over again. It poured out. I hit Send half an hour after I put fingers to keys.

It was still too early to call the East Coast to talk business, so I sent off a few work-related e-mails. I touched base with the kids—told them where I had hid extra money. My e-mail pinged. One of the Riverdale Goddess's fans left a comment. Feedback! It made me deliriously happy to know real, live people were out there, getting with the Goddess.

Thank you, RG [that's what friends called the Goddess], *for having the courage to write. When you let go of the craving for society's acceptance, you can have so much more in life. We have to fight the pain of full-out loving. The world doesn't welcome that. If I had buckets of the tears I cried for the self-loathing, from feelings of rejection and dissatisfaction over not having "him," they would flood Central Park. . . . I'm coming back into my own now, quite late in the game. Just like you, I'm finding myself on a massage table through one-way touch. I'm so glad I found you, Kate.*

There was nothing to do but thank her. Another ping. Someone else chimed in. Then another. The blog was a hive of opinion and response this morning. I expected some reaction to the DK post—it was edgy—but this was unprecedented for me.

I couldn't figure it out, so I checked the Google analytics. Hot damn. Readership spiked from a few hundred to thousands in thirty-six hours. It had to be a mistake. I investigated further and discovered that a celebrity blogger, a self-anointed arbiter of the blogosphere, had pronounced my "sex" blog too hip for words. One entry from her and "The Riverdale Goddess," playing for months in the ether sandbox, became an overnight center stage sensation.

This was better than dark chocolate. Almost. The comments were cascading in. People got it. I wasn't alone. I had the balls to say what so many people felt just below the socially acceptable surface about who's on top, power and surrender, masculine and feminine energies.

It was so thrilling that I ran back up to the room to tell my roomies, but Beth and Markus were still conked out.

"Beth, get up." I shook her until she showed a sign of life.

"Wassup?" She was narcotized. I made coffee in the room and handed it to her.

"Beth, honey, listen. I'm out at practice visits with Bob until this afternoon. Then he and Michael are coming over to do their session. They're gonna need a solid three hours here and we sure don't want to walk in on that. So I'll call you when I'm close to the hotel and we'll meet in the lobby and we'll get you a dress for tonight. I know exactly where to go for it. It's *the* place for your leather needs."

Beth rolled her eyes. "I thought it was all about the rubber?"

"That too, honey."

By the time I showered and dried my hair, my mind was caught up in the schedule of doctors we were pitching for support. One scone later, I was feeling pretty good. Highballing it across the sunlit Golden Gate Bridge to Marin with Bob behind the wheel, I was a happy blogging success.

Bob chatted away. "Michael is totally stoked for the Tiger," he said. "Me too." He floored the Chevy Malibu and said, "By the way, that was some blog this morning. You got some cojones on you, girl."

"There's no point if it's not honest," I answered.

"It certainly is honest. The stuff about your weight? You're going to help a million people struggling with body image. I'm proud of you."

"Bob, you can't imagine what that means to me," I sniffled, getting all emotional over his approval. "How long until we get to our first stop? I need to pee."

"You always need to pee. I have to remember to build in pit-stop time for any trip with you," Bob said.

An eternity later, we dragged our asses back to the city. We were both on fertility overload, talked out and pooped. He dropped me off at the hotel and I promised him privacy for his session. "Have fun, kiddo."

"We will," he shouted as he gunned it, leaving skid marks in his wake.

Beth was in the lobby, impatience written all over her face. Jeez.

"So let me get this straight," Beth started in. "I would take you and Markus to the Leather Fairies and you'd both be wearing leashes and collars. Markus would be my toy and *you,* missy, you would not speak or go anywhere without *my* permission. You are my slave?"

"That would be about right," I said, stifling a yawn, mining for any nugget of energy.

"I do like this. You do not get to talk? You both do what I say?"

"That's right."

Beth's eyes lit up. She was taking to being a "top" a little too easily. She was a natural dom dame. After thirty-five years of close friendship, there was something new between us.

"Let's get me a latex dress. Now!"

I jumped up, saluted, and held the door open for the walk to Madame S.

Once inside, Beth went on a fetish rampage. It was fascinating to witness this side of her. Despite "Celebrating the Body Erotic" together, we had no sexual interest in each other. Yet here we were, playing in unknown territory. Beth, obviously, was attracted to BD/SM. It was fun being in this sexual space with her, watching her vamp it up in different outfits, trying on different roles. It was like playing kinky Barbie dolls.

She came out in a thigh-skimming, nearly see-through, skin-tight shiny black latex and rubber minidress with garters. It left nothing to the imagination, hugging every curve and dip. Her ass looked great. With stockings and smokin' red pumps, Beth was a knockout.

"If I may, mistress, that's the one." She yipped and gave me a hug.

"Don't you want something?"

"Of course I do, but I have enough clothes. A girl can never have too many toys. I wanted to take you to Good Vibrations. It's a sex toy institution."

"I'm tired," Beth whined. "I wanna go back to the hotel."

"It's only five minutes away and you absolutely have to see their antique vibrator museum. I swear some of them look like Black & Decker power drills."

An hour later, we left Good Vibrations with something more up-to-date and lightweight than the Miracle Ball-Grip Massager, which looked more like a bowling ball than a vibrator.

We schlepped our bags back in time to grab a drink with Markus, who was exhilarated after his session with Bob and Michael. By then it was time to retreat to the room for a full-on game of dress-up. An unseemly amount of hair spray and makeup later, we were ready for our close-up. Beth's scarlet lips and gelled hair were magnificent. If I say so myself, I was ravishing if oxygen-starved in my corset. Markus put a kilt over the tiger stripes we painted on his chest, back, and bubble butt. My God, we were spectacular. I put on my collar and handed the leash to Beth. Markus did likewise. She grinned like an idiot.

We covered up as best we could, which wasn't quite enough. The doorman got an eyeful and said, "Don't you three look fantastic!"

I blushed, Beth stammered, and Markus pulled himself up straighter. He oozed confidence. San Francisco had become his home away from home during his Sexological Body Work certification course. He had tons of friends and was no stranger to the city's underground BD/SM world.

He shepherded us to a small tavern, where they ate and I watched. The corset was the best cheat-free diet ever. An hour later, we were in a taxi on the way to the Leather Fairies annual ball, our first invitation-only BD/SM play party.

Chapter Thirty-Seven

Long Live Love in Leather

The taxi screeched to a halt in front of an elegant town house somewhere off Folsom, where everything sexy seemed to happen. We were giddy with our own sophistication. My God, we were having a real live adventure. Beth and I were like thirteen-year-old middle school truants sneaking into a college party, pretending we belonged but nervous that we'd be found out.

"This is so cool." Beth pinched my arm the way she did whenever she did naughty things. I pinched her back. She slapped my hand and gave my leash a sharp tug. "Watch it. I'm in charge."

Blech. "Yes, mistress. Is this going to make Kevin jealous? You gonna tell him?"

She gave an extra, totally unnecessary pull and led the rest of the way up the stairs to the entry.

"This'll probably make him hot," Beth snickered.

Markus had already pushed the bell and was pawing the ground impatiently. Just as Beth and I made it to the top, a man in a crew cut, a little black sheath, high heels, and smoky eye makeup threw open the door. He was stunning and utterly unself-conscious. His strange beauty took me by surprise. The Leather Fairies were all about gender flexing and queer expression in the context of power and surrender. Markus, in his red-hot tiger stripes, did arrange this, after all.

"May I have your names, please?" Our greeter's resonant voice had an imperious twang. When he found us on his list, his lined face broke into a broad smile. "Welcome to Leather Fairies. You're going to adore us. And may I say, you look gorgeous." He couldn't peel his eyes away from Markus. Beth and I might as well have been invisible. "Yummy."

We walked through the foyer and came into a small dungeon play area equipped with a St. Andrew's cross (aka a flogging post), a spanking bench, and other BD/SM essentials. Beth's eyes were sparkling dangerously. My stomach gave an excited flutter. Markus dutifully handed Beth his leash and told her that before she could boss us about and set us up with playmates, we had to participate in the ritual "heart circle" that opened each monthly Leather Fairies party.

We joined about forty people in a circle and held hands. We ranged in age from maybe twenty-five to eighty, with bodies fit and not so fit, beautiful and taut, pear-shaped and saggy, cantaloupe round and beanpole thin. Like the three of us, some were dressed in fetish regalia, and others came to play in nothing more exotic than T-shirts and jeans. I took a long breath into the ritual safe space we were all creating and it felt like coming home. I loved this.

We welcomed the four directions—the east, the west, the north, and the south, as familiar by now as Daka Rock. Beth and I exchanged glances and smiled conspiratorially. We were as far away from peanut butter and jelly as we could have ever wished.

A "priestess" in her fifties passed around lettuce seeds so each of us could symbolically plant an intention in a pot of soil. She asked us to bless each other's tiny seeds as we tenderly pushed them into the earth. I was so engrossed and so filled with the love in that room, I didn't take in the full measure of our leader until we were concluding. She was a stunner, with long blond-gray hair and a soft skirt from which a black strap-on peeked with her every move. My eyes almost popped out of my head. At the risk of being gauche, I poked Beth. "Get a loada that."

"Shhh. We're in a ritual here," she whispered back. After a final group hug, the priestess gave us permission to go play. The experienced Fairies peeled off, and Beth led Markus and me by our leashes and instructed us to observe and learn.

All around us scenes were unfolding. A dark-haired older woman with pigtails who was dressed in a schoolgirl outfit was being flogged with playful intensity by a young man. She played with her master. She goaded him on, lifting her skirt or shirt, and laughing. She was gifted and experienced. In fact, the whole room was filled with old leather hands, people who were devoted to a flavor of power and surrender that was born out of their shared quest for spiritual connection. Some of them were world-famous artists in their own right. I'd never witnessed such play. It was spectacular.

Then I spied a sixtyish man in a kilt with a gray mustache and beard. He was using a bullwhip with exquisite accuracy on a woman about his age. She wore nothing but jeans and a black leather harness that left her back, breasts, and pierced nipples exposed. No words passed between them, but their eyes said everything. I caught the glint of their wedding rings. They were married, so married, and probably for a long time. The intimacy between them was yummy to watch.

I was fascinated by them. I was fascinated by him. I was aroused. The room was pulsating. The sounds and scents of play and sexual energy were so big there was no room for anything else. I kept watching the man in the kilt. Would he play with me? What would that be like? How would it feel if he said yes? How would it feel if he said no?

As I watched them, a sudden longing pierced my heart. I was shocked by the man's resemblance to Gavin. My God, I *am* powerfully attracted to my husband. Left to my own devices, I'd buy the same pair of shoes over and over. Here I was, spending time and resources exploring myself in ways that were once unimaginable, playing with people who were handsome, maybe even gorgeous. Yet, when I tuned into my own desire, it was an older man with an imperfect body, a bald head, and facial hair that I wanted. Gavin in a kilt wielding a bullwhip. I wanted him to dominate me. Riveted, I watched this Leather Fairies husband and wife and it flooded me with envy. They made room in their marriage for an outside spark to breathe and burst into a flame. I wanted that, too. At home. A geyser of sadness blew. Gavin's refusal to continue exploring with me made me want to weep. I could see for the first time what was sexually possible within the bonds of matrimony. The evidence was right in front of me.

We got back to the Queen Anne with only a couple of hours left to pack and get to the airport. We raced like lunatics, checked in, and waited for another two hours. I was exhausted, agitated, and generally upset. My libido was in overdrive after years of coasting. My heart was fighting off wave after wave of grief and melancholy. I didn't want to leave San Francisco.

I could see a life there, a different kind of life than the one I had in Riverdale. I understood that I was vibrating from my sexual-exploration marathon. I understood that this wasn't real, everyday life. But I wanted it to be. I knew I needed to "process my adventures."

Process, my ass. I was sick of introspection. These experiences touched a place beyond reason and I didn't want to go back to living my life in neutral. Resentment about the limitations of my "real" life was making me miserable. This wasn't part of my grand plan.

I just wanted to sit and cry.

It felt lousy going back to the relentless demands of my job, my family, and, most of all, my husband who had flipped the Off switch on our sexual growth together. I wanted—no, needed—him to be awake and alive.

On an impulse, I decided to call Gavin. Maybe some contact would throw the switch back to On. I needed to do something to feel connected.

"Honey, I'm at the airport."

"Great." I could tell he was looking forward to seeing me.

"Gavin . . . I went to a party last night. It was with Leather Fairies, a bunch of people who get together for a kind of spiritual BD/SM play. People were every age and every shape. Some have been playing together for twenty-five years! It was so interesting and sexy." I stopped just long enough to inhale.

"Honey, there was a couple there, a married couple, and they were having such a wonderful time together. I was so jealous. I want that with you. I want to be able to go out and explore with you. I want you, not someone else. This man there? He was the sexiest man in the room to me. He was bald with a goatee like yours. He wasn't ripped or perfect or young. This man, he reminded me so much of you and he was the one that I wanted."

"Ah-huh."

"Ah-huh? Ah-huh what?"

"Ah-huh. I don't know about any of this. I did try it with you and Markus. It just didn't do it for me. But I hear how much you want this, so I'm not saying definitely no. I understand what you're asking. Pamela. I love you. And I want to make you happy. But in this area, we have different desires.

"I'm not saying that I'm not willing to give it another go. But we don't always like the same things in the same way. We've been through this."

Gavin said he'd think about it, but I knew he wouldn't. I could feel my generator shut down.

All I could do was weep. This was overwhelming him. I got that. And he'd been so great, giving me so much freedom. I married a really unusual and wonderful man. But I wanted Gavin in a kilt. I wanted him to be a little bit edgy and sexy with the wonderful twinkle in his eye that he got after he had two beers.

Was I going to spend my life in sessions and workshops in order to meet my needs? In order to stay married? Would it be enough? It was enough up until now. But what about tomorrow?

It wasn't as if I could put my genie back in the bottle. This feeling coursing through my body was too good. I was too alive.

If I couldn't bring Gavin along, at the very least I wanted a sex-positive life in NYC. What I discovered in San Francisco was how much I loved leather play and the unique spirituality of that city's BD/SM community. If it existed in San Francisco, I figured it had to exist in New York City, too. And if it didn't, then I had to create it. My first step was to learn more.

Chapter Thirty-Eight
Goddess Lost

I'D GOTTEN USED to the sensual Technicolor of San Francisco. New York City was nothing but black-and-white. I needed and wanted more integration in my life. For now, the only balm for my longing was to pour my desire into my blog, often writing while Gavin slept with his head in my lap. One early spring night, frustration got the better of me. He'd been snoring away next to me as I put the finishing touches on RG's latest entry. I shook him awake and told him I was lonely. He said he understood that was a bad thing. "I'll try harder," he said, and went right back to sleep.

I studied his face as his mouth twitched into a dream smile. At least one of us was having a good time. I thought about my predicament. Gavin was attracted just like I was to dominant and submissive energies. I knew because I had found a well-thumbed edition of *The Story of O* in his dresser drawer.

I wanted my husband to be my top and my playmate. I wanted him to bust out of the old mold and become the puzzle master, the man who could fit all my pieces together into one whole work of art. I was okay with the plain vanilla of our marriage. I just didn't want it all the time. I needed him to break out of his damn box already. I didn't want to be lonely with him anymore.

So I went online. Now that I knew what I was looking for, it took no time to find like-minded people. It was a bigger and more robust community than I could have ever imagined. There were Listservs, monthly gatherings at restaurants called "Munches," play parties, workshops, and conventions. This was a different animal than "the Body Electric" and the serious pursuit of sexual spiritual healing. The groups I was finding in New York were much more recreational and hetero. I was elated. I'd found the perfect way to introduce Gavin into this world: dinner and a beer.

Subtle me, I made reservations for us to attend a local "Munch" and then to go to Paddles (the last public BD/SM club in the city) for a panel discussion about committed couples negotiating the kink scene. I dressed as sexy as I could for my husband, given that we were going to a perfectly respectable restaurant. I was an understated sex goddess in a provocative, form-fitting lace blouse, long black skirt, and tall leather boots.

We sat down to dinner at the back table of a Greek diner in Chelsea with ten other people, all of them perky and alive with possibility. Gavin sat slumped over, his shoulders curved so far I could have zipped them together in front of his chest

"Gavin," I said, trying to bring him to life, "did you know Ned sitting across from you loves sailing, too? He's almost as crazy about boats as you are." I was trying to find the way to engage him, to show him that he was still on safe ground.

He hardly acknowledged that I'd said a word, burying whatever response he had in his beer. I couldn't budge him. It felt like the other men were circling me like vultures after fresh meat, but Gavin didn't seem to notice. He was positively surly and withdrawn.

My spirit was sinking, but I refused to give up. I was hoping that by hearing the other couples slated to speak at the Paddles "educational forum," Gavin would be comfortable enough to give it a go. The club set up an area with about one hundred bridge chairs and a small stage for the panel. It was packed.

"Look around, honey. Everyone looks just like us. Not a corset in the room," I said, hoping he wouldn't notice the senior citizen in the baby-doll dress and bonnet. Gavin didn't even grunt. I bit back on the disappointment, because it *was* so ordinary. There wasn't a trace of the delicious San Francisco airy-fairy, "set your spiritual intention" atmosphere that I'd come to love. For me, this work was all about the healing alchemy of sexuality and spirituality. On the other hand, this was my city, my home, and I was grateful to find this place and this community.

The three-couple panel jumped onto the stage.

"See, Gavin? I told you. Normal." I directed his attention to the two couples who looked like Wal-Mart shoppers in no-name jeans. Nothing threatening. The third couple was a different story.

They identified as a "switch" couple, which meant they took turns topping each other.

"We want to bring a female submissive into our relationship. We want to share," said Kathy, a strikingly pretty woman of no more than twenty-eight or twenty-nine.

"Kathy's bisexual, and we thought it might be great to have a submissive woman in the house so she could explore her full sexuality with me in the picture," said Frank, an equally exotic thirty-something with black hair and smoldering eyes. "We could both top her. I'd really get off on that."

I poked Gavin. "Oooh, I wonder if I could apply for the job," I joked. Gavin didn't see the humor. He had stopped breathing.

Next came Gina and Jim, two dominants who shared a submissive. Then Shelly and Marvin from Long Island explained, "We like to go out and get the shit kicked out of us. Then we go home, have milk and cookies, and go to bed!"

Each couple had different tastes, but they all agreed that extramarital intercourse was off-limits.

I leaned over and whispered to Gavin, "You see, honey, they may be kinky, but they've got boundaries." As I heard myself, I started laughing. It all seemed so outlandish when I wasn't in San Francisco. Where were the Tibetan singing bowls?

As Gavin writhed, I cooed and flirted with my man. In a desperate attempt to save an unrelentingly awful evening, I pulled a collar out of my pocketbook and offered it to him. "Would you like to put this around my neck? You know, it means you're staking your claim."

"I staked my claim over two decades ago. This is just not my scene. This is your world, not mine. I wouldn't know what to do with you here, how to act, or anything," Gavin said in a defeated voice. "I can't top you."

He made a beeline for the nearest exit. I gathered up my things, trying to blink back the tears as I followed him out. I had miscalculated. I expected touchy-feely couples stuff and this was Kink Survival 101, practical and raw. I was at a loss. I'd tried everything I could think of to tell Gavin what I'd found and who I was becoming. A couples session with Markus. Books. Tapes. Workshop offers. Weekend getaway options. And now this.

My frustration and despair were at a near boil. I knew I was supposed to be gentle with him. I was supposed to tenderly lead him into my world. But it was like dragging a big burlap sack of bricks. I snapped. I had had enough. I was tired of all the yanking, pulling, and lugging.

"There's no hope for us!" I yelled as we marched into the parking lot. I couldn't believe I was behaving like a crazed harpy, but I couldn't stop. "I want a complete marriage! I want to be with someone who is my match. I can't do plain vanilla anymore. I just can't!"

"Why can't you be happy with vanilla? What's wrong with vanilla?" Gavin was anguished. I immediately regretted my words. I was being a creep.

"Vanilla is fine. But I don't always want vanilla. Sometimes I like chocolate swirl, sprinkles, and a cherry. . . . "

I turned away and walked to the opposite end of the parking lot, where I'd left my car. He'd driven here straight from work. It made me sad that I was so relieved to be driving home alone. I couldn't turn off my brain. I ranted and fulminated and ruminated. Could it be just as simple as the weariness of a longtime marriage? Maybe twenty-five years is too long to expect to be with one human being and have "hot" anything. Maybe I did need playmates who weren't my husband. Maybe I could never be one integrated person with anyone. Maybe I was still too big. I felt lost.

I needed to cry. Again.

Chapter Thirty-Nine

Who Makes the Rules, Anyway?

GAVIN BEAT ME home. He was in bed and asleep when I came in. That was fine with me. The lights were on in the boys' room. Andrew had popped in for the weekend.

"Time to shut it down," I hollered, uncharacteristically churlish. "Andrew! Ben! It's two a.m. Turn the computers off now."

"What's up with you?" Ben asked, poking his head around the door. His LCD-glazed eyes were more curious than concerned. "You know, Mom, we're not children anymore."

"You will always be my children. It's late. Go to sleep."

Ben's head disappeared, their door closed. Motherly duty done. I didn't know if they turned in or not, but I at least had the illusion of solitude. I needed some space to unload the roiling mix of thoughts and emotions that threatened to blow a hole in the top of my head.

From comments on my blog, I knew that I'd struck a chord that resonated wildly with people facing loneliness in their long-term monogamous marriages. I wasn't alone in my struggle. It was comforting to me to discover that other men and women loved their life partners as much as I loved Gavin. I didn't want to leave and neither did they. Yet on some level, we were unfulfilled. All of us were looking for more, seeking greater intimacy in our relationships. We were thirsting for more eroticism in our lives. They were just like I was when I started on this life trip—too frightened to do something about it, too frightened to do nothing. I used to be scared that I didn't have any desire left. They were scared about that, too. Now that I knew I had an abundance of erotic juice, I was terrified I'd never get to express it fully in one place.

I had swallowed the "happily ever after" marriage fairy tale hook, line, and sinker. I bought the story that if I was completely honest with my husband, my newfound desire would become the fairy dust that would make the sexuality in my marriage sparkle again. Bullshit. I've always known, deep in my own heart, that this past year was about me, not Gavin. This was about uncorking the bottled-up pieces of my soul, gathering them up and loving them. It was about letting go of the shame surrounding my desires, my body, my place in the world. If I was big and hungry, then so be it. Sure, I wished Gavin could have come along, but it wasn't in his nature. It wasn't *his* desire. I had to let go.

I got into my old T-shirt and crawled into the bed next to Gavin. His back was to me and I reciprocated. It was unsettling, and unhappily momentous. In twenty-five years, we had never slept back-to-back. I counted sheep and dropped off. When I woke up at my usual five a.m., there I was, wrapped around him, like always. The comfort of him flooded me.

He is my rock, my life's blood. I don't know if my heart would pump the same way without him. So he doesn't make my thighs radiate heat like he did when I was seventeen. A quarter of a century later, his touch does something less—and more. He loves me so deeply that he's willing to do things that he would never have done on his own in a million years. He does them because I ask him to. Because he says I excite him like no one and nothing else. There is security in our love. It's so complete and accepting, it moves me to tears when I let it.

He moaned, feeling my flesh next to his. I whispered in his ear, "Give me what no one else can give me. Let me feel your tongue between my legs. Let me feel you deep inside me."

I didn't have to invite him twice. Gavin was there for me, pleasuring me and bringing me to a lovely climax. I climbed astride him and rode. I looked down on his sweet face. He was so happy and content. This was precious. It was a part of what we are.

In that moment, I stumbled on a truth. What Gavin and I do together is the sex of our marriage. Our connubial bed has never been a place of the extended touch that I'd come to enjoy, need, and crave from the hands of my Sacred Intimates. It never was the spicy edge to which DK brought me. In our bed, I may never get lost in the sensual dreamscape that I'd discovered through the gift of one-way touch. But I still loved it—and it was just as important to me. This place—next to Gavin.

And isn't that how it sometimes goes? Just when I felt like I could not take one more minute—when I wanted to run away more than anything in the world—here I was making love to my husband. What I had learned is that it is often on that edge of pain that the most beautiful releases can happen. I reached for my husband's mouth and kissed him. Perhaps it is through persistence, the doggedly stubborn ability to stay, where the magic lies.

Epilogue

Now, that's what I call a happy ending. And it was. Except that it was just the beginning. All sorts of things happened after I rediscovered my husband's delicious embrace. Markus became a good friend after graduating me from his practice. Hank is still my Sacred Intimate. And DK? Well, that's another story. He became the man that tops me to this day.

The rest of my life, however, didn't go quite as smoothly. I got hauled before the organization's "unofficial" tribunal after Bob and Bitsy got scared that my blog would expose me, my organization, and maybe them to a "sex" scandal. They kept repeating, "Do you know what would happen if anyone found out the Riverdale Goddess was you?" I fought back—"I have no shame about anything I've done"—but they wore me down with veiled threats of professional ruin. They were going to out me before I was ready. I had two kids to feed and put through school. Not to mention that I loved my organization and giving it up was unthinkable. My family and my work were my twin pillars. I couldn't do anything to jeopardize the welfare of either. I caved.

They put me on kinky probation. But I didn't take well to the muzzle. (I never did like ball gags.)

I took down my anonymous blog, saved my job and my kids' tuition, and promptly thought about how I could sneak a new blog to life. I felt rebellious. I wanted to get back what I had lost. I became "The Renegade Goddess."

Unfortunately, I couldn't keep my big mouth shut. What a shock! After a great three-month run, I got snagged and my board friends officially defriended me. One might say my resignation as executive director wasn't entirely voluntary. It was messy, and occasionally I still get heart palpitations when I think about it.

I got the news that my "situation" was resolved and read the accompanying press release about my cheerful departure for greener pastures when I was in San Francisco practicing surrender. The beat, after all, does go on.

It's still thumping. I mean, once I saw how much better all parts of my life could be when I embraced my big, sensual, sexual side, there was no going back. I'd come too far toward being shameless, which is my code word for uncorking untapped desire, to withdraw into hiding. There were so many more cliffs to jump off. And I did.

Best of all, more and more people were telling me I wasn't alone. I just had to get the conversation rolling. So I outed myself. Remember the "scarlet letter" that scared me so much? It didn't take long for me to get used to it, and I started wearing it proudly. Did you know that red goes with almost everything? Once I felt brave enough to use my real name for my real life, everyone I talked to seemed to be grappling with their own untapped desires and their own shame. It made me wonder if being sexually alive meant having to suffer the judgment of others—personally or professionally—just because some of us dare to want to feel sexually whole. As long as what we're doing is safe and consensual between adults—then I say, screw suffering. Screw shame.

Pleasure is a much better place to grow from. Sure, there are consequences, but from my perspective, it's worth it.

Does that make me a sex radical? Nah! I'm still a pretty ordinary, ambitious, family-loving, housework-avoiding, diet-flunking everyday woman. Talk about liberation. I love being that overamped, chubby Betty Crocker in stilettos. Just shameless.

Acknowledgments

THIS IS A book about a part of my life that was not without consequences. I could not have lived it, or written it, without an incredible group of people who believed in me, supported me, and loved me through it all. My husband, known as "Gavin" in these pages, is a true love warrior who has stood by me with a fearless courageousness that has known no limits. My kids have put up with having an "out of the box" mother—and have never stopped cheering me on and making me laugh. You boys are my heart. My incredible mother, Roz, and my invincible sister, Tracey, are the original "shameless" women, and without them I might not have had the courage. I am one of the lucky ones who have had incredible role models in living life out loud.

I met Anne Adams, my cowriter, years ago when she interviewed me for the *New York Times*. Who knew that a simple interview would create an incredible friendship and collaboration? Whether the topic was fertility or a woman's right to know and own her sexuality, Anne has held my hand. She did more than help me shape my original blogs into a book—she provided hours of free psychotherapy. Without Anne, there would be no book—and no sanity.

It was Anne who introduced me to my fearless agent: Linda Loewenthal from David Black Literary Agency. She brought the faith and the belief that this book was important for all women. I will be forever grateful for her friendship and guidance. Linda lit the way to my editor, Colin Dickerman at Rodale Books. I fell in love with Colin the minute I met him—and I knew he was the one. And he was. Thank you, Colin. Props as well to Gena Smith, for her editorial insights and hand-holding!

I am also very grateful to the Rodale publicity team: Aly Mostel, Yelena Nesbit, and Sasha Smith, and to Goldberg McDuffie, Megan Beatie, and Liza Lucas.

For my Martini Gang and "Inside List" friends who read every word over and over again: Thank you for making sure that I never gave up. We did it and the drinks are on me. I love you. My BFF, Lisa Rosenthal, who is often the first person that I talk to in the morning—and the last one before I go to sleep at night. I can't imagine life without you.

And then there are the men—my teachers and my beloveds. Markus, my "pilot light man"; Hank, who taught me to speak desire; and DK, who remains the riverbank. There have been so many loving arms that have held me and taught me: Don Shewey, Brian Swager, David Cates, Mark Bednar, Joseph Aldo, Susan Isaacs, Alex Jade, Paul Barber, Joseph Kramer, Christine Fawley, Al Waddell, and Ellen Heed. My gratitude and love know no bounds. You helped change my life.

I can't forget Dave Kreiner, MD, for letting me be exactly who I am.

And last, but not least—for being my Knights in Shining Armor—Scott Browning Gilly, Esq., and my brother, Mark Sokoloff, Esq., for keeping my shameless ass safe. I will always be grateful.

BOCA RATON PUBLIC LIBRARY, FLORIDA
3 3656 0556419 6